T0256134

Handbook

Statistics and Data Management
A Practical Guide for Orthopaedic Surgeons

Dirk Stengel
Mohit Bhandari
Beate Hanson

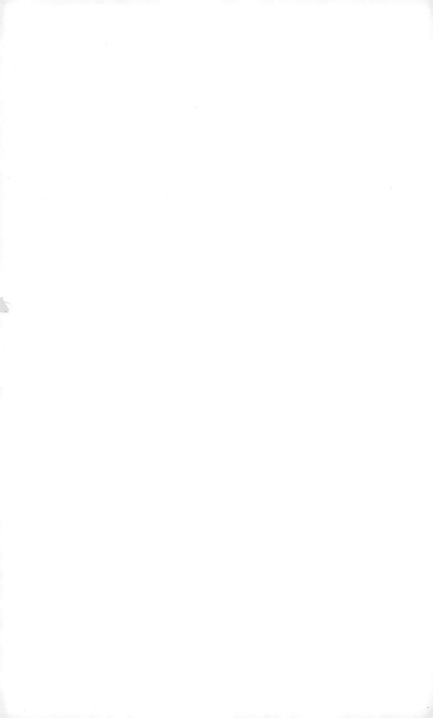

Handbook

Statistics and Data Management

A Practical Guide for Orthopaedic Surgeons

Dirk Stengel
Mohit Bhandari
Beate Hanson

 Thieme

Layout and typesetting: nougat GmbH, CH-4056 Basel

Library of Congress Cataloging-in-Publication Data is available from the publisher.

Copyright © 2009 by AO Publishing, Switzerland, Clavadelerstrasse, CH-7270 Davos Platz
Distribution by Georg Thieme Verlag, Rüdigerstrasse 14, DE-70469 Stuttgart and
Thieme New York, 333 Seventh Avenue, US-New York, NY 10001

Printed in Switzerland.
ISBN 978-3-13-152881-0

Table of contents

I   Introduction

Dear reader

We, the editors, authors, and all who contributed to this book, appreciate that, in addition to your daily commitment to patient care, you decided to spend extra time and efforts for clinical research. This will definitely make health care a little better, and this book may assist you in the difficult balancing act.

Applying new technologies, presenting your experience, and, of course, thinking of your current practice in the light of new evidence, needs some understanding of clinical research methodology. Your job is to save lives and limbs, and you are doing that perfectly—nobody wants you to become a statistician for a reasonable and clear evaluation of your results. But we need to share a common language, and reach consensus on basic scientific principles.

In fact, studies usually do not fail because of too little use of inference tests, but sloppy planning and inappropriate use of statistics. Data are vulnerable and need attention and diligent care. Spending more time in the beginning will spare time in the long run. Think of the variables you are really interested in, how they can be gathered, stored, processed, and analyzed. Regard statistics as a vehicle to generate and communicate information.

This is not a textbook, but a brief guidance for clinical research practice. It aims at bridging the different points of view of statisticians and clinicians, but does not replace personal meetings and discussions between both professions at the earliest step of a clinical study. Cooperation is vital. Talk. Argue, if necessary. Share opinions, and let your counterpart benefit from your specific expertise.

We hope that you find this book enjoyable, easy to read and understand, and helpful for improving your research skills. Let us know if we got the point.

Dirk Stengel
Mohit Bhandari
Beate Hanson

II Foreword

Sapere aude! (dare to know)   *Immanuel Kant, 1784*

Whether you love or hate statistics, you need it for clinical decision making, for counseling patients and their relatives, and to argue with those who decide which health care interventions will appear or remain on the market, or even in your hospital. You need statistical knowledge to make your way through the immense and ever-growing body of scientific literature, and, of course, to plan and conduct your own research. Research is an integral part of being a doctor—historically, today, and, far more important, tomorrow. As an orthopaedic or trauma surgeon, you offer a precious good—your skills and your commitment to your patients and the society. Sharing both your expertise and skepticism with the clinical and scientific community is important to bring this discipline forward. Take the helm, and participate in research actively.

The "Handbook of Statistics and Data Management" is obviously not another textbook about statistics. The authors, experts from both a methodological and a clinical point of view, wanted to be brief and concise, spoon-feeding you with the essential knowledge about numerical information, study designs, data storage, and analysis. This book is neither exhaustive nor complete; it just fits better into your daily business. You will probably agree that a book like this was not available to orthopaedic and trauma surgeons before.

Me, the editors, and the authors hope that it will help you to sort and focus your ideas when setting up a clinical study, and to understand why certain information should be expressed in this or that fashion, how data should be compiled, analyzed, and presented. It will help you to negotiate with your statistician—one of the most important persons you have to contact early during study planning. He will probably be amazed that you can express your specific problem in the common language of science—in numbers. And your colleagues will definitely congratulate you that you are able to retranslate numbers in a more important language—the clinical impact of research findings, and the benefit to our patients.

David L Helfet

III   Contributors

Editors

Dirk Stengel, MD, PhD, MSc
Head of the Center for Clinical Research
Department of Trauma and Orthopaedics
Unfallkrankenhaus Berlin
Warener Strasse 7
12683 Berlin, Germany

Mohit Bhandari, MD, MSc, FRCS
McMasters University
Epidemiology and Orthopaedics
1200 Main Street West
Hamilton, Ontario, L8N 3Z5, Canada

Beate Hanson, MD, MPH
Director of AO Clinical Investigation and Documentation
AO Clinical Investigation and Documentation
Stettbachstrasse 6
8600 Dübendorf, Switzerland

Authors

Laurent Audigé, PD Dr (DVM, PhD)
Group leader Methodology
AO Clinical Investigation and Documentation
Stettbachstrasse 6
8600 Dübendorf, Switzerland

Kai Bauwens, MD
Senior Consultant Surgeon
Unfallkrankenhaus Berlin
Department of Trauma and Orthopaedics
Warener Strasse 7
12683 Berlin, Germany

Mohit Bhandari, MD, MSc, FRCS
McMasters University
Epidemiology and Orthopaedics
1200 Main Street West
Hamilton, Ontario, L8N 3Z5, Canada

Richard E Buckley, MD, FRCSC
Head Division of Orthopaedic Trauma
University of Calgary
Foothills Medical Center
Department of Surgery
AC 144A
1403 29th Street NW
Calgary, Alberta, T2N 2T9, Canada

Axel Ekkernkamp, MD, PhD
Director
Unfallkrankenhaus Berlin
Department of Trauma and Orthopaedics
Warener Strasse 7
12683 Berlin, Germany
Professor of Surgery
Department of Trauma and Orthopaedics
University Hospital of Greifswald
Sauerbruchstrasse
17475 Greifswald, Germany

Norbert P Haas, Prof Dr med
Charité Universitätsmedizin Berlin
Centrum für Muskuloskeletale Chirurgie
Campus Virchow-Klinikum
Augustenburger Platz 1
13353 Berlin, Germany

David L Helfet, MD, MBCHB
Professor of Orthopaedic Surgery
Cornell University Medical College
535 East 70th Street
New York, 10021, USA

Thomas Kohlmann, PhD
Professor and Director
Institut für Community Medicine
Abteilung Methoden der Community Medicine
Walter Rathenau Strasse 48
17487 Greifswald, Germany

Peter Martus, PhD
Professor and Director
Charité Universitätsmedizin Berlin
Campus Benjamin Franklin
Institut für Medizinische Informatik,
Biometrie und Epidemiologie
Hindenburgdamm 30
12200 Berlin, Germany

Jörn Moock, PhD
Institut für Community Medicine
Abteilung Methoden der Community Medicine
Walter Rathenau Strasse 48
17487 Greifswald, Germany

Dirk Stengel, MD, PhD, MSc
Head of the Center for Clinical Research
Department of Trauma and Orthopaedics
Unfallkrankenhaus Berlin
Warener Strasse 7
12683 Berlin, Germany

Michael Suk, MD, ID, MPH
Assistant Professor
University of Florida
Director, Orthopaedic Trauma Service
College of Medicine Jacksonville
655 West Eight Street, 2nd Floor ACC
Jacksonville, FL 32209, USA

1 About numbers

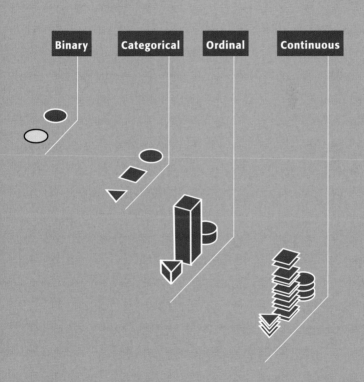

Binary

Categorical

Ordinal

Continuous

1 About numbers

1 About numbers

1 Introduction

Numbers can be our friends or foes. They can express information very precisely, or may sometimes put us on the wrong track. Without some knowledge of the anatomy and physiology of numbers, it is almost impossible to conduct meaningful research. The aim of this chapter, therefore, is to introduce you to the proper selection and interpretation of numbers required to transport and distribute your ideas.

To ease communication with your colleagues, you have surely already acquired a personal dictionary of acronyms, synonyms, and abbreviations. As a surgeon dealing with musculoskeletal injuries and diseases you are familiar with terms like ED, OR, CT, MRI, ExFix, or ORIF (emergency department, operating room, computed tomography, magnetic resonance imaging, external fixator, open reduction and internal fixation). Correct use of these terms facilitates communication and forms an important element of your professionalism. You may, however, meet with problems when doing business elsewhere without adapting your vocabulary. Medical language and terminology can be confusing, and similar terms may have very different meanings.

Numbers have a fascinating attribute—they are unequivocally recognized as such by clinicians and researchers, other healthcare professionals, your patients, and everybody, regardless of their background, affiliation, or nationality. The language of numbers is global—so it is the perfect language of science. You may use numbers to encrypt the tons of information you collect about your patients in daily practice, to describe their demographic profile and individual risks, and the results of your treatment. However, using the correct code and choosing the appropriate numbers is essential to compile, handle, and process clinical information.

> *The key to a successful research project is to translate*
> *distinct clinical information into the correct numerical vehicles.*
> *The key to evidence-based practice is to retranslate*
> *the information encoded in numbers into clinical language.*

2 Numbers to describe individual patient characteristics

Information about patient characteristics can be expressed by numbers in one of four major classes of data:
- Binary (or dichotomous)
- Categorical
- Ordinal
- Continuous

Binary (dichotomous) data

The simplest type of information imaginable may be stored in the form of data variables having only two possible categories, such as yes or no, one or zero, male or female, left or right, the presence or absence of a disease or an injury. Such variables are called binary or dichotomous. Although categories may be expressed in words, the data may be stored as numbers or binary information (Fig 1-1). Chapter 5 "How to analyze your data", chapter 6 "Present your data", and cross-tables will focus on the utility of binary information.

a

Age	Male gender*
23	1
35	1
42	0
52	1
65	0

* Male gender:
true = 1
false = 0

b

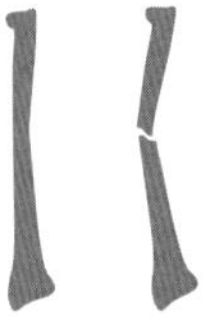

intact   broken

Fig 1-1a–b
a Example of categories expressed in numbers.
b Example of categories expressed in words.

Categorical data

A fracture of the radial bone may occur in its proximal, mid-, and distal third, which has implications on the treatment, but not necessarily on the outcome. The anatomical classification is value-free, which is the key characteristic of categorical data (Fig 1-2). Another typical example is the pattern of blood types (A, B, AB, and 0). Numbers attached to these categories do not have an intrinsic value and are only used to help store the data and run analysis.

---

a
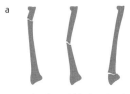

proximal   midshaft   distal

b   *A variable called "fracture localization" may be stored as:*

1 = proximal
2 = midshaft
3 = distal

Fig 1-2a–b
a   Characteristic of the categorical data is that it is value-free.
b   Categorical data can be numbered according to the requirements.

Ordinal data

There are, however, categories which can be placed in distinct order (ie, category B is worse than category A). This type of data is called ordinal data (Fig 1-3). Within the Müller AO Classification of Fractures in Long Bones, a complex, intraarticular fracture with multiple fragments and alteration of the cartilage layer (type C) has a worse functional prognosis than an extraarticular type A fracture. Other examples are the American Society of Anesthesiologists (ASA) risk classification scheme (ASA I–V) or the Gustilo-Anderson grading of open fractures.

Ordinal data variables very often have a limited number of possible categories such as in the later clinical grading systems. These variables are also said to be noninterval because the intervals between adjacent categories (often expressing prognostic information) may not be equal. The difference between type C and type B fractures may not be the same as that between type B and type A fractures.

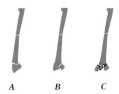

Fig 1-3   Ordinal data are categorized in a distinct order.

Continuous data

Finally, data variables may be used to store information from counts or measures that, in principle, can take infinity of values within clinically plausible ranges. If you are interested in the treatment of osteoporotic fractures, the T-Score obtained by a dual energy x-ray absorptiometry (DEXA) is a good example of a continuous measure with obvious prognostic impact (Fig 1-4).

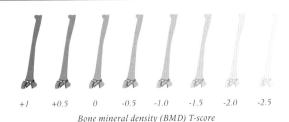

Bone mineral density (BMD) T-score

Fig 1-4   The T-score obtained by a DEXA is a good example of continuous measure with obvious prognostic impact.

Counts are integers

Some continuous data can simply be counted.

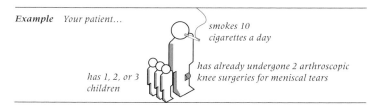

Example   *Your patient...*

smokes 10 cigarettes a day

has already undergone 2 arthroscopic knee surgeries for meniscal tears

has 1, 2, or 3 children

Counts are said to be integers, which means that they are expressed as number of units (nobody has 1.4 children or presents with 2.7 fractures). In practice, integers have often only a limited number of plausible values to choose from (eg, a person has only a limited number of children or fractures in a life time).

Most basic characteristics of an individual are best described by integer values, eg, age, height, weight, etc:
• You are stabilizing the grade I open femoral shaft fracture of a 49-year-old male using an intramedullary nail.
• During operation, he requires 2 units of packed red blood.
• It takes you 60 minutes to complete the procedure.

Measures are intrinsically nonintegers

Some continuous data require measuring.

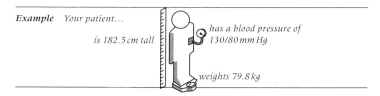

Example   *Your patient...*

has a blood pressure of 130/80 mm Hg

is 182.5 cm tall

weights 79.8 kg

Measures are intrinsically nonintegers because they can take infinity of values expressed by the use of decimals. They can be expressed as integers if they are directly recorded or rounded to their unit (eg, when age is expressed as 49 years instead of 49.2 years).

Data variables stored as numbers thus contain information of different complexity. The complexity of information increases from binary to continuous values. They may describe:
- A certain fact with valuation (someone has 2 or 5 children)
- A certain fact without valuation (someone wears a blue, white, or red jacket)
- A scenario with prognostic impact (someone needs 2 or 5 units of packed red blood)
- Or distinguish between two different clinical situations (a patient with a femoral fracture has a blood pressure of 60/35 mm Hg or 130/80 mm Hg)

3   Numbers to describe the attributes of a group of patients

3.1 Patient listing versus summary statistics

According to Albert Einstein's famous quote, everything should be made as simple as possible, but not simpler. You spend much time collecting data of varying complexity so, in conducting your analysis, do not hastily rip them to pieces, nor squeeze them into rough classes or categories. In doing so, you may miss subtle, but important associations.

> *Whenever possible, utilize the full range of information provided by your data.*

In a scientific article, and with a small sample size of 20 patients, you may have two different ways (Table 1-1 and Table 1-2) of presenting the demographics of your patients.

> *Tabulate individual patient data—you will mostly use integer values (Table 1-1).*

Strengths   Tabulating individual patient data provides the most comprehensive overview of the studied population. It allows presentation of extreme cases (eg, the 84-year-old female), a view of associations between variables, and to recalculate summary statistics.

Limitations   Tabulating individual cases may only be possible with small sample sizes and a limited list of measured items. As a rule of thumb, 20–30 patients represent the upper limit.

Patient-ID	Gender	Age (years)	Duration of surgery (minutes)	Units of packed red blood
1	male	18	91	0
2	female	25	49	0
3	male	49	68	1
4	male	58	71	2
5	male	71	63	5
6	female	50	55	3
7	female	40	109	0
8	male	31	45	0
9	male	69	60	0
10	male	54	67	1
11	male	58	90	1
12	male	82	84	2
13	male	19	56	4
14	female	47	79	0
15	male	31	64	0
16	female	59	102	0
17	male	67	61	3
18	male	69	53	2
19	male	73	50	1
20	female	84	47	1

Table 1-1   Patient listing with individual patient data and integer values.

*Tabulate summary statistics—you will often come up with nonintegers (*Table 1-2*).*

Characteristic	
Gender (n)	
Male	14
Female	6
Mean age (years)	52.7
Mean duration of surgery (minutes)	68.2
Mean number of units of packed red blood	1.3

Table 1-2 Summary statistics with a group of patients resulting in nonintegers.

In a series of 20 patients (14 males, 6 females) with grade II open femoral shaft fractures, the mean age was 52.7 years. On average, 1.3 units of packed red blood were transfused, and the mean duration of surgery was 68.2 minutes.

Strengths This type of presentation allows easy reference to your patient profile. The reader can quickly decide whether the studied population fits into their practice, and can compare these findings to those from other investigations.

Limitations The table may obscure interesting individual cases, which are often helpful for clinical problem solving in difficult or rare situations.

It is important that you express clinical information in the most clinically relevant data form and round continuous variables appropriately, for example, how many digits should be measured and presented after the decimal point? Think of the patient's age—do you feel it makes sense to provide a mean age of 59.698745 years? Does it provide more necessary information than a mean age of 59.7 years?

Increasing the number of decimal places suggests a precision in measurement, which is neither achieved in a biological system, nor useful for interpreting the data.

Values with more than two decimal places are rarely needed.

Many periodicals demand four decimal places for *P* values (which definitely makes sense).

3.2 Simplification of data

Occasionally, it can be useful and necessary to reduce the complexity of information. This may happen when you generate groups of subjects from continuous data in a clinical study, or when you combine categories of categorical data.

Strengths   Working with data in their original format retains their full informational content. Native data may describe your population or the variability of treatment results better than simplified categories.

Limitations   Especially with continuous measures, small units can produce spurious, clinically irrelevant associations between the variables of interest.

Consider the categorization of continuous data

Older patients may have more severely impaired shoulder function after fractures of the proximal humerus than younger subjects.

In terms of the Constant-Murley score, the average difference between the fractured and the healthy side is 0.25% for any additional year. In other words, a 66-year-old patient will have a shoulder function that is 0.25% worse than that of a 65-year-old patient, who has a 0.25% worse function than a 64-year-old patient and so on (Fig 1-5a). A difference of 0.25% may be clinically meaningless and difficult to communicate. Thus, thinking in larger categories clarifies the message: Patients between 66 and 75 years come up with a difference in the Constant-Murley score that is 3% worse than in patients between 55 and 65 years (Fig 1-5b).

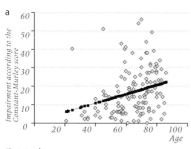
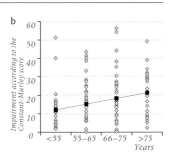

Fig 1-5a–b
a Native data may describe more details.
b Categories clarify the message.

Appropriate categories

Building appropriate categories is a trade-off between clinical and statistical reasoning.

Example *You may be interested whether patients with grade III A open fractures have poorer functional outcomes than those with grade I open fractures. However, your group of 60 patients with open fractures may comprise the following fractures:*

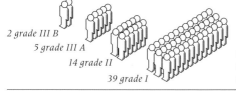

2 grade III B
  5 grade III A
    14 grade II
      39 grade I

In this case, it can be necessary to rethink your original question.

You might consider grouping patients with grade II, III A, and III B fractures to generate two samples of reasonable size.

When data is ordinal, as in our open fracture grading example, grouping should be done only between adjacent categories. It would make no sense to combine grade I with grade III injuries to compare them with grade II injuries.

Helpful tools to split continuous data into subgroups of equal size are the so-called percentiles. For most purposes, you will need only two of them:

- 50% percentile (known as the median)
- 25% and 75% percentile (or first or third quartile)

As suggested by their name, they cut a sample in half or in quarters (Fig 1-6).

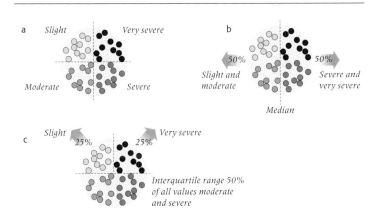

Fig 1-6a–c   40 patients with multiple injuries, graded according to the injury severity score (ISS).
a   The percentiles present natural thresholds which separate your data into groups of similar size.
b   Dividing your sample along the median will generate two groups of equal size. 20 patients with slight and moderate injuries, and another 20 patients with severe and very severe injuries.
c   The central portion (or the sirloin) of your data is described by the interquartile range (IQR). The IQR encompasses those 50% of patients with moderate or severe injuries. This data body has two appendices on either side, including 25% patients each with less or more severe injuries.

A word of caution: In our example the words "slight", "moderate", "severe", and "very severe" apply only to the data split according to percentiles. They imply an ordinal data structure of the simplified data. In different studies, the same injury severity score (ISS) may be labeled differently because the percentiles will likely differ.

Categorization of values is only possible in a top-down fashion. A continuous measure may be summed up in certain categories, and categories may even be dichotomized, but not the other way around.

The format of your data should fit with your measuring instruments (how precise and exact are they?) and your clinical problem.

4 Mean versus median

When providing summary statistics, you will need to decide whether the mean or median of continuous data should be presented.

Although everybody is keen on normal distribution, most data are skewed in the one or the other direction. If you are recruiting patients onto a clinical study, you will not enroll toddlers. Thus, the age distribution in such a sample will be oriented toward older patients (in the easterly direction). Most patients in your emergency department will have a systolic blood pressure of 120 mm Hg, with few presenting almost killing values of 200 mm Hg or higher. In this case, your data cloud will be geared toward lower values (in the westerly direction).

The median has interesting characteristics. Since it always cuts a sample in exact two halves, it remains robust against extreme values and outliers. While the median does not care for data skewness, the mean does.

The mean, or sample average, is susceptible to even small disturbances at the edges of your sample of values (Fig 1-7).

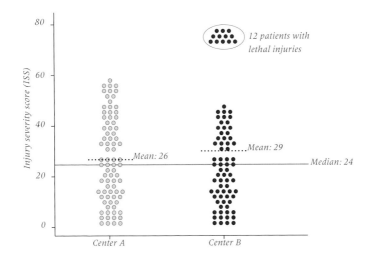

Fig 1-7   Consider our study, the injury severity of patients admitted to two different trauma centers is investigated.
- Center B took care of a higher proportion of more severely injured patients.
- However, note that a similar number of patients (50%) with an ISS up to 24 were treated at both institutions.
- So the median, cutting the sample in halves, is 24 in either group. Reporting only the median would obscure the obvious imbalance.
- Providing of the mean ISS fully illustrates the difference between the two cohorts (26 in Center A, and 29 in Center B)

The median is robust against skewed distributions.
It is the metric of choice in small sample sizes (eg, between
5 and 20 patients). It does not tell the full story about your
patient sample, since it obscures extreme values.

The mean is vulnerable to skewed distributions. It is the metric of choice when using continuous data in larger cohorts and when the data distribution is not severely skewed. Because of its susceptibility to data in the top and bottom of your sample, it provides hints on the underlying distribution and allows for calculating average differences.

5   Proportions, rates, odds, risks, and ratios

You have now acquired useful knowledge of the key features of numbers and values. However, when targeting a clinical problem in a research project, you may not only be interested in absolute values, but rates, proportions, odds and risks, as well as ratios. It is often necessary to illustrate the relationship between two items. There is confusion with these terms, so we need some taxonomy.

Rates
A rate expresses the relationship between two variables with different units (like miles per hour, or beats per second).
Typical rates:
- The incidence rate
- The number of first events of a certain disease
- Injury per number of person-years
- You may also trade-off costs and complications (eg, 10,000 US$ per surgical site infection).

Proportions and risks
Proportions and risks have very similar characteristics, and the difference in naming is mainly related to the event of interest. Both describe the relationship between two variables with similar units like the number of patients with a certain event or condition among all studied patients. One may provide numerators and denominators (eg, 1/1,000), or a percentage (eg, 0.1%).

There is some overlap (and hence often confusion) between these measures.

There are two different ways of expressing frequency of events. Fig 1-8a describes how many events have occurred in a certain number of patients (here: 4 of 10) and in a certain interval of observation. Fig 1-8b shows that each of these patients had a different time of exposure (expressed by the "time tail"). Note that there are very different patterns in the relationship between exposure time (for example, the duration of antibiotic treatment for joint infections) and events (for example, recurrent infection):

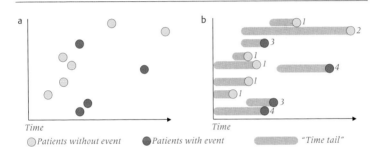

Fig 1-8a–b
a   Certain number of patients—certain interval of observation (4/10).
b   Each patient with different time of exposure.
    1   Short exposure time—without event (these patients may have dropped from the analysis because they could no longer be reached).
    2   Long exposure time—without an event.
    3   Short exposure time—with event (in case of antibiotic treatment, those patients would represent clear treatment failures).
    4   Long exposure time—with event.

You may also be interested in observing patients without an event for a much longer time. Thus, their time tail overhauls the current assessment, and will add to the next follow-up.

Imagine you follow 1,000 patients during a full year (= 1,000 patient-years) and observe just one event of a condition.

The cumulative incidence of this condition can be expressed as:
Rate = 1 per 1,000 patient-years
Risk = 1/1,000 or 0.1%

Both measures give the same result when all patients are followed during the entire period of observation, but this almost never happens (Fig 1-8).

If, let us say, 20% of patients were observed only half of the time (eg, lost after 6 months), 200 patients would account for half of the patient-years, which means 100 patient-years.

While the risk would not change with 1,000 patients at the start of the observation period, the rate would be 1 per 900 patient-years.

For practical reasons, we may be comfortable with this very basic distinction. You will find, however, that rates are often expressed as percentages or, what one often calls rates (eg, mortality rate or complication rate), may be in fact risks.

Odds
Odds are defined as the likelihood of a thing occuring rather than not occuring. They differ from a risk in that the denominator does not include the patients with the condition. If 5 in 100 patients had a certain exposure, the corresponding odds is 5:95 or 0.053.

Ratios
Ratios are used to describe the relative effect of a certain intervention compared to another.
There are two main types of ratios:
• Risk ratio (RR)
• Odds ratio (OR)
These ratios are intrinsically tied to the underlying study design, so it is necessary to go a little into details of study design.

Study design

The association between a certain intervention or exposure and the target outcome can be investigated on two different timelines (Fig 1-9):

- Retrospectively: using available information from patient records and hospital charts
- Prospectively: by beginning with data collection as soon as patients enter the institution and following them up for a specified interval

The line of vision from the exposure to the event or from the event to the exposure forms further two design options.

Cohort study

If you set out to compare the bone healing rates after fixation of distal tibia fractures by intramedullary nails compared to interlocking plates, you will think of the following chronology—in the typical order of a cohort study:

1) Sampling your patients
2) Assigning them to one or the other fixation method
3) Obtaining x-rays after 6 months to determine fracture consolidation

The major characteristic of a cohort study is that you start with a patient sample and two or more different interventions to explore a certain outcome. In other words, at the beginning of the cohort study, you are fully aware of the treatment assignment of your patients, but not of their outcomes.

A cohort study can be carried out prospectively or retrospectively.

In a prospective cohort study, all new patients admitted to your department will form your study sample. After treatment, they will be followed-up and reexamined after a predefined period of time, and the outcome of interest evaluated (Fig 1-9a).

In a retrospective cohort study, you start with identifying patients that had been treated at your institution, eg, in the hospital's administrative data base, or the operating theatre logs. By reviewing the outpatients' charts, and/or contacting patients by mail or phone, you retrospectively assess whether they reached the outcome under investigation (Fig 1-9b).

Obviously, the prospective study is more time-consuming, but will provide more reliable data than the retrospective study. With a prospective design all physical findings and questions of interest, and supplemental information like x-rays, can be obtained at a predefined time, and in a standardized fashion. Datasets are likely to be complete after you have finished your follow-up procedures.

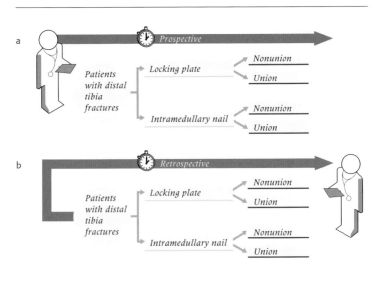

Fig 1-9a–b   Cohort studies start with intervention and end with <u>outcomes</u>.

In the retrospective setting, many data are immediately available from the medical documentation, and the interval between treatment and outcome may have already passed—thus, your information is ready to use. However, eligible subjects may not have attended their appointed outpatient visits, or cannot remember whether and when the outcome of interest had occurred (eg, for instance, when the time they resumed their daily activities). This can be a significant source of bias.

In a prospective cohort study (and only in a prospective cohort study) the individual treatment can be assigned by chance (which makes up the randomized controlled trial).

Case-control study
Cohort studies are suitable if you have sufficient numbers of patients with a common disease or injury. However, if you are interested in whether a certain exposure, such as smoking, has any influence on a rare outcome (eg, epidural infection after dorsoventral stabilization of a lumbar spine fracture), a cohort study is not the appropriate design. You may spend the rest of your life waiting for enough patients with the rare targeted outcome in a prospective cohort study. You may also go crazy by scanning thousands of patient records to identify smokers and nonsmokers who underwent spine surgery and did or did not develop epidural infection.

In this situation, you may start with collecting all epidural infections first, without knowing whether these patients are smokers or not. You may then identify patients with similar characteristics (same gender, age, body mass index, and so on) who underwent the same surgery with uneventful recovery. Finally, you identify how many smokers and nonsmokers were in either group. This approach characterizes the case-control study. Case-control studies are always retrospective.

At the beginning of the case-control study, you are fully aware of the outcome of your patients, but not of their treatment assignment or certain risk factors like smoking (Fig 1-9c).

There is much confusion with the definition of case-control studies, especially in the orthopaedic literature. Please keep in mind, that the term "case" always refers to patients who reached a certain endpoint (eg, nonunion), whereas "control" always indicates those who did not reach that endpoint (eg, those who united uneventfully). "Case" and "control" do not describe the treatments under investigation (eg, intramedullary nails versus locking plates).

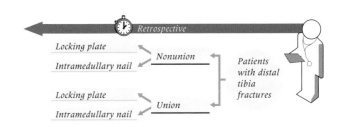

Fig 1-9c   Case-control studies start with <u>outcomes</u> and end with intervention.

In a cohort study, the line of vision is directed from the intervention towards the event.

In a case-control study, the line of vision goes from the event back to the exposure or intervention.

Each study type has its appropriate ratio metric. In a cohort study, the relative effect can be expressed as a risk ratio (also called relative risk) or an odds ratio. In a case-control study, only odds ratios must be used.

> *Odds ratios (OR) can be used in both cohort and case-control studies. The risk ratio (relative risk) (RR) is exclusively reserved to the cohort study.*

Imagine an archetypical cohort study in orthopaedic surgery with the aim of finding out whether, compared to conservative treatment, suturing of the Achilles tendon decreases the risk of reruptures.

You may be lucky to enroll 100 patients in either arm (well, you may be even luckier if you are able to assign them randomly to treatment groups...). After 6 months and tireless efforts to achieve complete follow-up, you come up with the 2×2 table (Table 1-3).

> *Suturing halves the risk of a rerupture compared to conservative management (Table 1-3a).*

Another way to look at the data is from a case-controlled prospective. Here you start with the event of interest (eg, rerupture).

> *Patients with a rerupture are twice likely to have had conservative rather than surgical treatment (Table 1-3b).*

| Treatment | Event | | |
	Rerupture	Healed uneventfully	Total
Suturing	4	96	100
Conservative	8	92	100
Total	12	188	200

	Suturing	Conservative
a Risk of rerupture	4/100 = 0.04 or **4%**	8/100 = 0.08 or **8%**
b RR compared to the alternative treatment	4%/8% = **0.5**	8%/4% = **2.0**
c Odds of having ondergone surgical treatment	4 : 8 = **0.5**	96 : 92 = **1.04**
d OR estimation	0.5/1.04 = **0.48**	1.04/0.5 = **2.09**

Table 1-3a–d   The source of the ratios is the cross-table.

a   The risk of rerupture after suturing is 4/100, or 4%. The risk of rerupture after conservative management is 8/100, or 8%.

b   The RR is simply the risk of rerupture in the suturing group, divided by the risk in the conservative group. This leads to 4% and 8% respectively = 0.5. (The RR of rerupture in the suturing group is 0.5 compared to that of the group with conservative management). Conservative treatment doubles the risk of rerupture compared to surgery (8%/4% = 2.0). (The RR of rerupture in the group with conservative management is 2.0 compared to the suturing group).

c   Of twelve patients with a rerupture, four have been treated surgically for an odds of 4 : 8 = 0.5. On the other hand, 96 of 188 patients with uneventful healing have been treated surgically giving an odds of 96 : 92 = 1.04.

d   Consequently, the OR is estimated at 0.5/1.04 = 0.48 or 1.04/0.5 = 2.09, respectively. Thus, patients with a rerupture were 2.09 more likely to have undergone nonsurgical rather than surgical treatment.

Beware that very often the OR is interpreted as if it was a risk ratio. One may say about the OR that "Achilles tendons undergoing conservative treatment have 2.09 times higher odds to rerupture compared to those undergoing surgery". The correct interpretation is that reruptured tendons were 2.09 more likely to have been treated nonoperatively.

> *Only when the targeted event is rare, the OR and RR*
> *are very similar and therefore the OR is a good approximation*
> *of the RR. Otherwise, interpretation errors may lead to a*
> *major overestimation of the strength of effect of an intervention*
> *(or any other exposure).*

OR and RR in a large trial
Thanks to the success of your study, you were awarded a research grant, and patients are keen on participating in a much larger trial. Again, your energy paid off in the complete follow-up of 1,000 patients each (congratulations!).

Whatever the reason, you still observed only 4 and 8 reruptures. This dramatically changes your absolute risks (4/1000 = 0.4%, and 8/1000 = 0.8%), and odds (4:996 = 0.0040, and 8:992 = 0.0081).

What happens with your ratios? The RR remains unchanged at 0.5 in favor of the suturing group or at 2.0 in disfavor of the conservative treatment group. The OR is getting closer and closer to the RR with the increasing rarity of events (Table 1-4).

Treatment	Event Rerupture	Healed uneventful	Total
Suturing	4	996	1000
Conservative	8	992	1000
Total	12	1988	2000

	Suturing	Conservative
Risk of rerupture	4/1000 = 0.004 or **0.4%**	8/1000 = 0.008 or **0.8%**
RR compared to alternative treatment	0.4%/0.8% = **0.5**	0.8%/0.4% = **2.0**
Odds of having undergone surgical treatment	4 : 8 = **0.5**	996 : 992 ≈ **1.00**
OR estimation	0.5/1.00 ≈ **0.5**	1.00/0.5 ≈ **2.00**

Table 1-4   The larger the trial the closer gets the OR to the RR.
The RR remains unchanged at 0.5 in favor of the suturing group or at 2.0 in disfavor of the conservative treatment group. The OR is getting closer and closer to the RR with the increasing rarity of events.

6   Risk difference and number needed to treat (NNT)

Perhaps the simplest, still most important and clinically relevant statistic to be calculated from the 2×2 table and risk estimates is the risk difference (RD). In our first Achilles tendon study example, the RD is $8\% - 4\% = 4\%$ (Table 1-3a). In other words: Suturing reduces the absolute risk of sustaining a rerupture of the Achilles tendon by 4% compared to conservative treatment.

The RD expresses the absolute effect of an intervention compared to its control.

A popular metric is the number needed to treat (NNT). The NNT describes how many patients must be treated with the experimental compared to the control treatment to avoid 1 additional event. The NNT is the inverse of the RD, or 1/RD. In the present example, the NNT is 1/4% = 25.

This means: 25 patients with a rupture of the Achilles tendon must undergo surgery rather than conservative treatment in order to avoid 1 extra event of a rerupture.

In our second Achilles tendon study example with increased sample sizes, the risk difference now is only 0.8%−0.4% = 0.4%, leading to a NNT of 1/0.4% = 250 (Table 1-3b).

The number needed to treat (NNT) is calculated at 1/RD and explains how many patients must be treated by intervention compared to the control treatment in order to avoid 1 extra target event.

Strengths   Absolute differences, as expressed by the RD and NNT, are indicators of the clinical value of a certain intervention. They disclose irrelevant treatment effects, regardless of large relative measures.

Limitations   In case of frequent conditions and large patient populations, small absolute differences may underestimate the importance of observations.

7   Summary

- Many characteristics of individuals can be counted and described by integer values, whereas measurements and summary statistics are expressed by nonintegers.

- Limit the number of decimal places to express appropriate data precision and clinical relevance.

- The four classes of data with increasing complexity are binary, categorical, ordinal, and continuous.

- If condensing complex data into categories, use percentiles (eg, quartiles) instead of arbitrary values.

- The median is more robust as the mean in skewed data distributions, and measures of data spread provide a good overview of the full range of data.

- The results of cohort studies can be expressed as risk ratios (RR) (also relative risks) or odds ratios (OR), while case-control studies demand OR. The OR approaches the RR only when studying rare events.

- The risk difference (RD) and number needed to treat (NNT) are further useful effect measures for clinical interpretation.

2 Errors and uncertainty

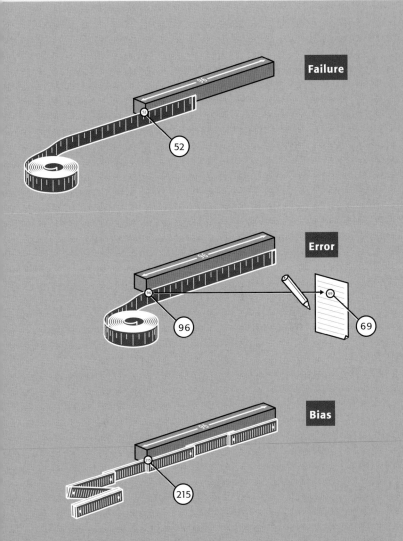

2 Errors and uncertainty

2 Errors and uncertainty

1 Introduction

Uncertainty makes life interesting and challenging. You may have worked out a well-structured plan for your day at the hospital or your private office, but this can be messed up within minutes because of sudden events or because you missed an appointment or task. This does not mean that your time was wasted. You may achieve very different, equally important results, make new discoveries, and enhance your knowledge because you followed a direction slightly different from that intended.

The same is true for a scientific experiment, whether it is laboratory or clinical. Uncertainty corresponds to the unexplained variability of observations. Forecasts and predictions (not only of weather) are susceptible to an enormous number of variables, and you never know if you considered all of them during the planning phase of your project. Of course, if any observation in biomedicine was entirely predictable, we would not need scientists anymore.

In clinical practice, you may have made a certain observation in a distinct setting for the first, second, and third time. This makes you believe a specific association or rule, but the fourth time you observe the exact opposite of what you had expected. Certain findings, though impressive and breathtaking, may occur simply by chance. The famous philosopher Karl Popper was of the opinion that a hypothesis cannot be proved due to the fact that we do not have access to an infinite amount of information.

2 Descriptions of uncertainty

2.1 Accuracy and precision

Uncertainty, variability, and error are integral parts of science. Unavoidable as they are, and in some instances desirable, they should be expressed and handled in a qualitative and quantitative manner.

We may be inclined to assume that a point estimate derived from a clinical study (eg, a change in functional scores, bone healing rates) reflects an absolute truth.

However, study findings represent a summary, aggregate, average, or extract from a sample of patients. On an individual basis, results may differ dramatically from subject to subject, or within a subject at different time points. To communicate information, we often need to abstract these results, and to abandon individual observations in favor of the sample mean.

> *All scientific work generates a likely range of observations that supports or weakens a theory, compatible or incompatible with a hypothesis.*

It is important to know how close the range of observations and the extreme values are to the average. Fig 2-1 illustrates this by a set of studies investigating quality of life after fracture treatment, using the physical component score (PCS) of the short-form 36 health survey (SF-36). This global measure of physical health is standardized to the population norm. The norm value is 50; values below that indicate a health status worse than the norm, values above indicate a health status better than the norm. Two studies came up with mean values of 50, but with very different distributions. We trust the estimate of a single study more if it is surrounded by many similar values and very few outliers, as in study 2.

> *The accuracy of an estimate is high, if it comes close to the truth, with many similar values and few outliers.*

It is also important to know whether the estimate is replicable, ie, if repeated studies come up with similar trends, or show a heterogeneous or random pattern. This refers to the precision of an estimate.

The precision of an estimate is high if repeated studies come up with similar trends.

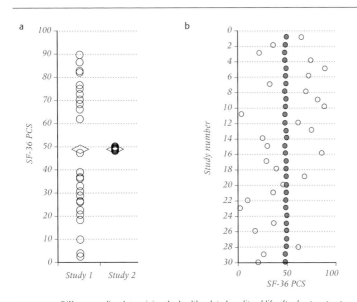

Fig 2-1a–b   Different studies determining the health-related quality of life after fracture treatment.
a   Studies 1 and 2 have similar mean values, indicating restoration of physical function to norm values. Study 1 has a wide distribution of values, making the estimate inaccurate. Study 2 shows high accuracy of the estimate because the distribution of values is narrow.
b   Thirty further studies, each of two different fracture treatments. Repeated studies indicated by a solid dot consistently come up with almost similar results in one treatment group. The precision of this treatment effect is high. In contrast, highly variable results are observed with studies in the other treatment group indicated by circles. It is uncertain whether an observation can be reproduced in a subsequent trial.

Imagine a new femoral nail intended to be inserted through the trochanteric tip. Fig 2-2 indicates the entry points achieved by four different surgeons during the first clinical trial of the new product.

Surgeon A created a series of entry points at the trochanteric tip quite close to each other. He achieved both high accuracy (low variability) and precision (in aiming the correct entry point).

Surgeon B inserted all nails through the trochanteric fossa. He achieved high precision, but low accuracy, since all insertions were made away from the correct entry point. There may be two different reasons for this: failure and systematic error, or bias. First, he may have not read the instruction manual and failed to use the implant correctly because he did not know how. Second, his usual access route and patient positioning may conflict with the tip entry. He may insert a nail through the fossa blindly, but still needs to adapt his technique to the new implant. Until he realizes this, the shape of the new rod may cause problems in the distal part of the femur and worse outcomes compared to the established implant—not because of inadequate hardware, but due to surgeon-related bias. The surgeon may also have mistakenly entered the nail through the fossa, despite having planned to target the tip.

Surgeon C attempted to enter the medullary canal through the trochanteric tip, but made drill holes within a larger area than surgeon A. On average, all nails may have been inserted accurately, but with low precision.

Finally, surgeon D requires the assistance of an experienced colleague, since all entry points were placed away from the correct site, and somewhere within the trochanteric fossa.

Situation B is critical and underlines the importance of bias. You may observe astonishingly high complication rates (such as distal cracks or malalignment), and conclude that the new implant requires improvement; however, the true reason for unfavorable outcomes must be looked for elsewhere.

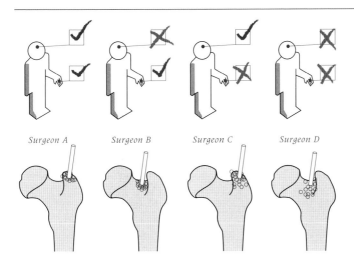

Fig 2-2   Entry points of a new tip-entry femoral nail achieved by four different surgeons.
Surgeon A: both high accuracy (low variability) and precision (in aiming the correct entry point).
Surgeon B: high precision, but low accuracy (all insertions away from the correct entry point).
Surgeon C: nails may have been inserted accurately, but with low precision.
Surgeon D: all entry points away from the correct side with high variability.

*Systematic error, or bias, should always be considered
as a likely explanation of unexpected findings.*

*Any investment to explore and minimize bias in a clinical
trial is valuable and pays off in the long run.*

*In a clinical study that compares two or more treatment
interventions, there is only one way to remove bias—
to randomly allocate patients to study arms.*

2.2 Randomization

There are many objections to randomized controlled trials (RCTs) in trauma and orthopaedic surgery, most of which are unfounded. If you have two treatments, and do not know which performs best in a typical clinical setting (eg, in a certain type of fracture), there is no easier and better way to do this than by an RCT.

Fractures of the distal tibia may be suitable for minimally invasive plate osteosynthesis and nailing. Imagine that you had performed ORIF by plate in 20 patients, and by nail fixation in the subsequent 20 patients, all of whom had similar fracture types. After 1 year, you observe nonunions in 1 and 5 patients, as shown in Table 2-1.

Unfortunately, although the patients' age, gender, and even the duration of surgery were well balanced, there were clearly more smokers in the nailing group. It is thus unclear whether the intervention or the smoking influenced the higher rate of nonunion.

You may now consider including only nonsmokers to avoid this bias. After 1 year, you now observe higher nonunion rates in the plating group. Unfortunately, two patients cheated you about their smoking habits, and another resumed smoking after years of abstinence shortly after discharge from the hospital. You also realized that there were an unequal number of diabetics in your study.

The list of potential confounders is almost endless, and can only contain those that are known and measurable. There may be distinct genetic factors that contribute to bone healing, but genetic profiling cannot be performed on a general basis.

Characteristics	Plate	Nail
Mean age, years (SD*)	34 (10)	35 (10)
Male : female	18 : 2	17 : 3
Duration of surgery, min (SD*)	94 (9)	99 (10)
Smokers	2 (10%)	10 (50%)
Nonunions	1 (5%)	5 (25%)

Table 2-1   Twenty patients treated in each treatment group. Number of nonunions related to different characteristics. Higher nonunion rate in the nailing group due to the smokers. It is unclear whether the intervention or the smoking influenced this result.

* SD = standard deviation

The randomized controlled trial (RCT) is the only design that avoids bias by equally distributing known and unknown risk factors between study groups.

The RCT generates treatment groups that are qualitatively (not necessarily quantitatively) comparable.

Since randomization makes study groups biologically similar, all differences in outcomes may be assigned to the intervention of interest, not to an imbalance in risk factors (bias).

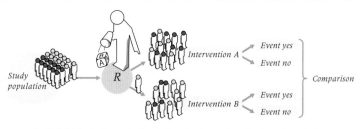

Fig 2-3 The RCT distributes known (yellow dots) and unknown (blue dots) equally to study arms. R = Randomized allocation

2.3 Types of error

You may have heard about type I (alpha) and type II (beta) errors. Understanding their meaning makes it much easier to plan a study, and to interpret its result. Since this is a handbook, not a textbook, put the following descriptions in your trial toolbox, and follow them wisely from the very beginning of your project. Both types of error must be specified together with your study hypothesis, and before starting patient recruitment.

Type I error (alpha error)

Beneficial and detrimental health effects can occur by chance, and may not be specifically associated with the treatment under investigation. Imagine you compare the new femoral nail with an established rod, and observe malalignment in 10% and 5% of all cases. A possible reason for this observation is bias by improper surgical technique, as described earlier. However, it may happen that you repeat the study, and find no difference in malalignment between the study groups, or even a 5% difference in favor of the new nail.

> *Patients must always accept a certain risk of undergoing a treatment that—although apparently effective in a clinical trial—may, in fact, be ineffective. This is the meaning of the type I error (alpha error).*

Of course, we want to set this error to the lowest possible value, because we do not want to expose our patients to an ineffective treatment. Type I errors of 5% are typically accepted, but this is only a convention. It means that a benefit of the new treatment over the control may be observed by chance in one of twenty hypothetical repeats. It also applies to the number of endpoints tested. If you strive for twenty different outcomes, you will observe a difference in one of them simply by chance.

The lower the risk of false-positive observations the lower is the type I error. You may set the type I error to 1% (which means only 1 in 100 tests will produce a positive finding by chance).

There is much confusion as to the meaning of the type I (alpha) error and the *P* value—and we must stress that (at least in theory) they are not the same. Unfortunately, the magical 5% threshold has evolved as a standard for both the type I error and *P*. Again, it is simply a convention, although a very reasonable one. The famous statistician Ronald A Fisher argued that, if only 1 in 20 experimental results may be assigned to chance, there is good reason to believe in the results, and a causal association between the intervention of interest and the observed outcome.

We cannot discuss the theoretical background and the history of these values in detail. However, you may find the following two explanations helpful:

> *The appropriate type I (alpha) error must be chosen before data collection, using sample size formulas or calculators. It equals the residual risk which you are willing to accept that a new treatment is wrongly regarded as effective, even though it is ineffective.*

> *The P value is generated by statistical test procedures after data collection, and indicates whether the observations are compatible with chance. The lower the P value, the lower the likelihood that chance is the best explanation for your findings.*

Type II error (beta error)

If all preclinical data of a new orthopaedic implant tend towards favorable results, the next step is to prove this in a clinical setting. However, as the risk of obtaining false-positive results, there is also a risk of missing an effect, ie, producing false-negative results.

> *Researchers must always accept a certain risk of missing a treatment effect. Even though an experiment reveals a difference between study groups, statistical testing may indicate a nonsignificant result. This is the meaning of the type II (beta) error.*

This risk can be minimized by increasing the sample size of a study. Nowadays, typical type II errors range between 10 and 20%, which again is a convention. It makes sense that type II errors are higher than type I errors. It is more dangerous to patients if a treatment is approved that is, in fact, ineffective, rather than to withhold a treatment because a study failed to demonstrate a difference to the standard of care.

The reciprocal of the type II error is the power of a study, a term you will be familiar with.

The statistical power (1–beta) describes the probability of a study to detect a distinct treatment effect.

Choosing appropriate type I and II errors is always a trade-off between safety concerns and feasibility. If you excessively lower the type I error in the best interest of your patients (for example, the residual probability that a new treatment is not effective is only .0000000001%), this will avoid almost any risk, but no new treatment will be available to them.

Aviation experts argue that it is theoretically possible to construct a failure-free commercial airplane, but that you would have to pay one million dollars for a domestic one-way ticket.

On the other hand, if you want to ascertain that even tiny differences between treatments will be detected with a 99.9999999999% chance, you will require an almost infinite number of patients.

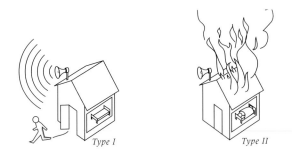

Fig 2-4   The type I error (alpha error) can be compared to a fire detector that raises alarm although it is not burning. The type II error (beta error) is the false-negative counterpart—it burns but the fire detector keeps silent.

2.4 Comparison and contrast

If you stabilize a fracture type A3 (according to the Müller AO Classification of Fractures in Long Bones) of the distal radius with a volar locking plate, and all patients show a good to excellent outcome, the next question must be: In comparison to what alternative: a T-plate, a Pi-plate, or an external fixation? Or even compared to conservative management?

The results of a study, and the outcomes observed with a certain intervention compete with those of other investigations and interventions. Only the comparison, the observation of a difference, or the similarity between two modalities reveals something about their value in health care.

> *Observations made in a single cohort of patients and with a single intervention are valuable in deciding whether the intervention works in principle, but only the comparison to another cohort of patients or to another intervention allows inferences to their effectiveness.*

Contrast is another important principle, and is the basis for quantitative measurements (Fig 2-5). A difference in a clinical study may be statistically significant, but clinically irrelevant. Statistical tests can be likened to a photo-processing software, and clinical expertise to our retina and visual cortex—we still need to interpret, before we believe, accept, or refuse a certain finding.

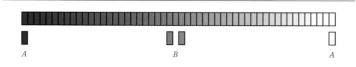

Fig 2-5   Contrasts in clinical studies can be understood as demonstrated in this color chart.
A It is clear that there is a difference between colors at the extreme left and right ends of the bar.
B The more we move our focus from the ends toward the center, the more we face difficulties distinguishing between the different shadings. Although there is still a measurable difference in brightness, it is no longer visually recognizable.

A scientific experiment rarely comes up with a black or white result, but a likely range of observations. The more the range of observations made with two different interventions overlap, the more the difference becomes undistinguishable. The greater the difference, the less likely that it disappears in a cloud of overlapping observations (Fig 2-6).

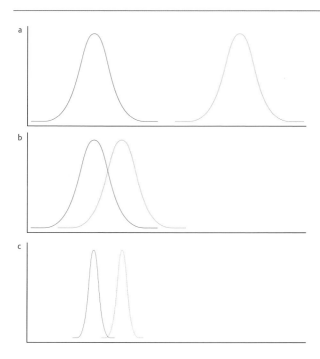

Fig 2-6a–c   A difference between two treatments will be recognized if the difference between mean values is quite large, and thus resistant against a wide distribution of values (a), or if the difference between means is small, but the distribution of values is narrow (c). If a difference in means is small, and the distribution of values is wide, effects are diluted and difficult to recognize (b).

3 Sources of variability

3.1 The measurement

If we repeat a certain measurement, eg, an x-ray of lower limbs of the same person under identical conditions, by the same radiologist, and at almost the same time, we can assume that variations are due to the measurement device. In our example, this would mean that there are sources of error somewhere within the technical process from the lens to the final image.

We cannot completely exclude that there is a short-term variation within the subject. For example, it may be possible that the position of the subject varies slightly, which may result in a difference of a few millimeters in the final evaluation. But these changes could be corrected by some calibration systems or they would have to be summarized under the measurement error.

3.2 The observer/reader

It is the aim of each measurement process to make the method independent of the observer. However, there are many reasons why measurements may be interpreted differently by different readers. With radiological images, experienced observers (in contrast to beginners) clearly differentiate between artifacts and true findings. A fracture may be differently classified by different observers, and if the severity of a fracture has prognostic implications, this will influence the interpretation of outcomes.

3.3 The subject

There might be changes of the "true" measurement value within one subject over time. If we only have one measurement per patient, these changes will contribute to the total variability seen in our sample. It may well be that each measurement would oscillate in the long term for one patient even though there is no trend toward larger or smaller values over time. Short-term variability might be reduced by multiple measurements, if possible.

3.4   The population

The final source of variability is different from others. Variability between subjects is a biological phenomenon. Populations demonstrate heterogeneity of subjects. This in itself might be the focus of interest in a study.

Different sources of variability possess a large impact on the practical aspects of a study. In summary, there exists undesired variability which we want to reduce as much as possible. Measurement error may be reduced by improving technical devices, observer variability by the training of observers and through independent reading, long-term variation within subjects by standardization of the measurement condition. However, since we cannot fully avoid measurement error, we need to know and to report its degree, and to respect this when interpreting our results.

4   Distributions

Values obtained in a clinical study always show a distinct distribution. They may be distributed symmetrically around the mean, or show certain peaks and tails. We need to know how data are distributed before we can decide the appropriate summary measure (see also chapter 1 "About numbers", subchapter 4 "Mean versus median"), whether statistical testing makes sense, and which type of test is suitable for statistical analysis.

> *Knowledge of the underlying distribution is the prerequisite for analyzing and reporting data.*

4.1   Normally distributed data

The typical bell shape of empirical data distribution is well known. From a theoretical point of view, we assume that data samples taken from a target population are normally distributed for the variable of interest. This theoretical distribution is an idealization of the true distribution in the target population.

The ideal bell curve with perfect symmetry is seldom found in real data, but in many cases, it is an approximation required for statistical testing.

The example shown in Fig 2-7 displays differences in disability of the arm, shoulder, and hand (DASH) questionnaire scores between baseline and 1-year follow-up assessments in patients with conservatively treated fractures of the proximal humerus. A null difference means that patients have fully recovered to their preinjury health status. Positive differences indicate worsening, whereas negative differences indicate improvement compared to baseline levels.

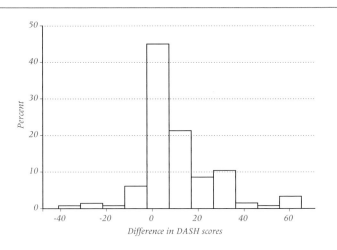

Fig 2-7   Differences in DASH scores between baseline and 1-year follow-up assessments in patients with conservatively treated fractures of the proximal humerus. The bell shape is not perfect, but many analysts would agree that, in this case, we could have used statistical methods for normally distributed data.

4.2 Skewed data

A bell-shape curve cannot be found with all variables of interest. When analyzing raw DASH scores after 1 year instead of differences to baseline values, we note a left-tailed data distribution of values, equating an exponential distribution. Most patients reported only slight impairments in shoulder function, and only few had severe problems (Fig 2-8).

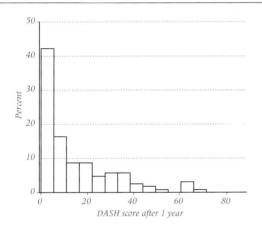

Fig 2-8   Raw DASH scores after 1 year.

4.3 Other distributions

There are many other data distributions. For example, if we are interested in success rates (eg, the rate of bone healings) or complications, data follow a binomial distribution. In case of very rare events, the so-called Poisson distribution applies. There are also complex, multimodal distributions with two or more peaks, such as the incidence rates of distal radius fractures that occur frequently in children, adolescents, and the elderly.

It is not necessary to know the exact mathematical formulas behind all distributions, but to keep in mind that they determine how to proceed with your data analysis. Thus, describe the underlying data distribution first (eg, by plotting a histogram), and use it as a guide for choosing the appropriate test strategy.

5 Standard deviation versus standard error

The two statistical parameters, standard error and standard deviation, are often mixed up. To make a long story short, it can be said that standard errors are used to calculate limits of confidence, whereas standard deviations serve to calculate normal ranges. This is demonstrated in the following theoretical example.

Example   *In the given example of functionally treated fractures of the proximal humerus, 127 patients were evaluated after 1 year for differences in DASH scores to baseline levels (see Fig 2-7). We obtain the following information on the data:*
  - *Mean = 10.2*
  - *Standard deviation = 16.5*
  - *Standard error = 1.5*

5.1 Standard deviation

The standard deviation (SD) is a measure of how the DASH differences vary within the population of 127 patients.

Example   *If data are normally distributed, we can derive a normal range for these differences by a very useful rule of thumb:*
  - *32% of the population are within the interval mean (10.2) ± one standard deviation (16.5).*
  - *95% of the population are within the interval mean (10.2) ± two standard deviations (2 × 16.5).*
  - *99.8% of the population are within the interval mean ± three standard deviations (3 × 16.5).*

This is illustrated in Fig 2-9. The differences in DASH scores are between -22.8 and 43.2 in about 95% of all patients.

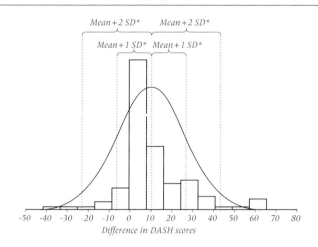

Fig 2-9   The mean and the standard deviation give information on data ranges, if they are distributed normally.

* SD = standard deviation

Standard deviations are excellent parameters to explain the variability of data, but only if they are normally distributed.

5.2 Standard error

What is then the meaning of standard errors? We could be satisfied with our study if we know the average DASH results, and their standard deviations. However, does this mean that, if you repeat the study, you will obtain the same results? Will the results apply to all patients you are going to study and treat in near future?

We need a measure of precision of our estimates. Intuitively, it should be clear that for this question, it is crucial that we know from how many patients our estimate has been derived. In fact, the precision of our estimate depends on two figures—the width of the normal range, and the number of patients in the study.

There is an easy way to transform normal ranges into so-called confidence intervals, and vice versa:

Width of confidence interval = width of normal range / $\sqrt{n}$
Width of normal range = width of confidence interval × $\sqrt{n}$
(n denotes the size of the sample)

Thus, if the normal range of the DASH difference in 127 patients has a width of ± 16.5, the confidence interval has a width of ± 16.5/$\sqrt{127}$ = 1.5. Assume that we double the sample size. Then the width of the confidence interval would be ± 16.5/$\sqrt{254}$ = 1.0.

As the name suggests, the confidence interval tells you how confident you can be that your results do not only apply to one single study, but will occur with high probability in another and with another cohort of patients.

The 95% confidence interval has emerged as one of the most important statistical measures in the scientific literature. It means that if you would repeat the study 100 times, you would observe values that are within the confidence interval in 95 of the times. In our example, the 95% confidence interval of the difference in DASH scores ranges from 7.3 to 13.1. Thus, in 100 studies, the mean difference in DASH will be somewhere between 7.3 and 13.1 in 95 studies.

The confidence limits are affected not so much by deviations from the normal distribution as by the normal ranges. The reason for this is that averages of measurements from different patients become more and more normally distributed even if the single measurement in the population is not.

We have tried hard to avoid formulas in this book, but you will find the next two a helpful. They represent the general method of how to calculate confidence intervals for means and proportions:

$$\text{Means } (\mu) \qquad \mu \pm 1.96 \times SD/\sqrt{n}$$

$$\text{Proportion } (p) \qquad p \pm 1.96 \times \sqrt{p \times (1\text{-}p)/n}$$

Note that the (approximate) standard errors for proportions and means are essentially the same. Further note that the formula for proportions becomes less accurate if the sample size n is small or if the observed proportions are near to zero or near to one.

6   Summary

- Uncertainty, variability, and error cannot be avoided in a scientific experiment. It is important to find appropriate ways of quantifying and expressing them.

- Heterogeneity across subjects in a population or a clinical study is often "normally" distributed.

- Describing the underlying distribution is an essential step before proceeding with data analysis.

- Standard deviations are very good parameters to explain the variability of data, but only if they are normally distributed.

- Confidence intervals describe the precision of estimates, and the probability of obtaining similar results in subsequent studies or groups of patients.

3 Outcome selection

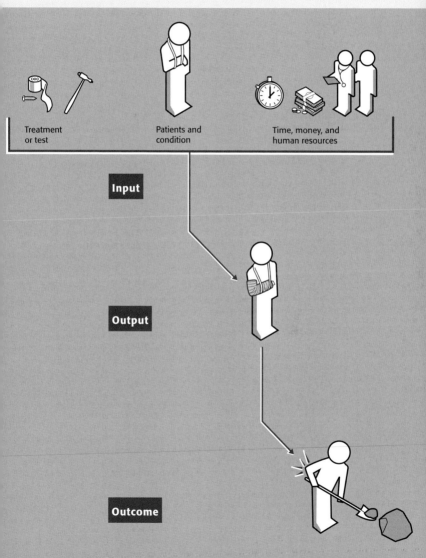

Treatment
or test

Patients and
condition

Time, money, and
human resources

Input

Output

Outcome

3 Outcome selection

3   Outcome selection

1   Introduction

In a scientific project, it should be clear at the very beginning which condition or intervention is to be studied, and also what type of endpoint you are aiming to achieve, to improve, or to modify. We have already stressed that all efforts must be made to formulate a precise, answerable study question, to organize your project around that question (taking care not to lose track), and to collect data that helps you answer that question.

In clinical research and care, always start by giving some input—an individual or a sample of patients who undergo a certain diagnostic test, or a surgical procedure. This inevitably generates costs. Other than purchasing the test kit, implant, drug, and so on, it requires time, personnel resources, and more to apply the intervention. A patient, however, may suffer inconvenience, pain, adverse events, and other risks and discomforts associated with the procedure. Add these puzzle pieces together, and as the ultimate result of the intervention under investigation, you may observe an output. Examples of outputs are an anatomically reduced intraarticular fracture, pain reduction after kyphoplasty, or the depiction of a meniscal tear by MRI scanning.

However, you will remember patients who do not stop complaining about pain despite perfect x-rays following ORIF of a pilon fracture, adjacent vertebral fractures in patients 1 year after kyphoplasty, and patients who underwent arthroscopic meniscal resection showing postoperative infection. This elucidates the difference between outputs and outcomes. Short-term measures of success (often called surrogate endpoints, such as radiographic findings or laboratory parameters) do not necessarily predict long-term outcome benefits. Outcome benefits are improved function, health-related quality of life, return to work, and social and leisure activities, or prolonged life. The cascade and hierarchy from inputs via outputs to outcomes is illustrated in Fig 3-1.

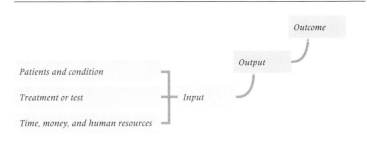

Fig 3-1 The trade-off between inputs, outputs, and outcomes.

Outputs are mainly surrogates of health status improvement, but must not reflect better patient outcomes.

Any clinical study should seek to trade-off inputs, outputs, and outcomes.

In health economy, an intervention is of added value, if either gain on outcome exceeds input, or similar outcome can be achieved with less input.

Regardless of discipline, medical professionals strive to improve aspects of patient health. It is necessary to have the means to quantify patient health status to ensure continued improvement of the standards of care. Instruments measuring changes in patient health over time, either as a result of an intervention or natural history, are termed outcome measures. Many outcome measures within orthopaedics are based on scoring systems. In clinical research, outcome scores are used to compare surgical techniques, prostheses, fixation methods, and types of perioperative care. They are also used for comparison between surgeons, departments, medical institutions, and countries. Postoperative outcomes can be assessed using a variety of measures including mortality, morbidity, clinical and radiological findings, postoperative complications, and health-related quality of life.

Health-related quality of life always includes a physical,
psychological, and social aspect.

Recently, there has been greater pressure on orthopaedic surgeons to evaluate the outcomes of their practice. Increased patient awareness and expectations, evidence-based medicine, and fiscal considerations are likely contributing factors. Yet, selecting an outcome instrument can prove to be challenging. In addition to having the necessary instruments available, a selection must be made; for example for the shoulder joint alone, there are nearly 30 outcomes instruments available.

As a result, clinicians often settle for a generic health status instrument such as the short-form health survey questionnaire with 36 questions (SF-36). Although general measures may be suitable for comparisons of health, a measure designed to be disease-specific will normally be more appropriate.

This chapter is intended to familiarize you with clinically relevant and methodologically sound measures of outcome, and to review techniques to improve the validity and reproducibility of study trial endpoints.

2   Validation of outcome measures

Before selecting a trial endpoint, the instruments available to measure that outcome must be considered. Therefore, it is necessary that orthopaedic surgeons are able to assess the quality of an instrument. A quality outcome instrument is one that has undergone the appropriate testing and has shown to be valid, reliable, and responsive (Fig 3-2).

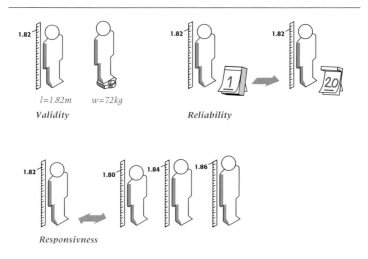

$l=1.82m$ $w=72kg$

Validity

Reliability

Responsivness

Fig 3-2   The three key components of a useful and accurate outcome measure. It must be valid, ie, it can measure precisely what it intends to measure. It must also be reliable, ie, given there is no change over time, it should come up with the same value after repeated measure. Finally, if there is change, the instrument should be able to detect this change (responsiveness).

Validity is simply the degree to which an instrument measures what it intends to measure.

Reliability reflects the consistency of measurements, that is the ability of an instrument to repeatedly measure in the same way.

Responsiveness represents an instrument's sensitivity to change as the status of the patient changes.

Validity and reliability can be distinguished with the help of the terms precision and accuracy explained in chapter 2 "Errors and uncertainty", Fig 2-2.

2.1   Validity

An instrument is said to have face validity if it appears to measure what it intended to measure. Outcome instruments are constructed to measure specific variables within a defined patient population and should only be considered valid for use in relation to that purpose. For instance, a validated measure of disability for patients with knee osteoarthritis following total knee arthroplasty cannot automatically be considered valid for use in patients with distal femoral fractures. To interpret the validity of an instrument, multiple concepts are considered. In orthopaedic literature these concepts include the notions of content, criterion, and construct validity (Fig 3-3).

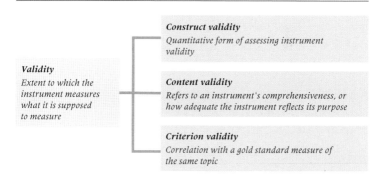

Validity
Extent to which the instrument measures what it is supposed to measure

Construct validity
Quantitative form of assessing instrument validity

Content validity
Refers to an instrument's comprehensiveness, or how adequate the instrument reflects its purpose

Criterion validity
Correlation with a gold standard measure of the same topic

Fig 3-3   The three different components of validity.

Content validity

Content validity reflects an instrument's comprehensiveness. It examines the ability of the instrument to measure all aspects of the condition for which it was designed. Generally, as the content of an instrument increases, the reliability decreases proportionately. This is very much comparable to diagnostic test research—only few tests are both highly sensitive and specific at the same time. With high sensitivity (or high content validity) you will probably not miss any patient having a certain disease (or any single aspect of the target condition). However, this is likely to be at the price of low specificity, or reliability—you might falsely diagnose healthy people as sick (or measure aspects that, in fact, have no meaning for the target condition).

Therefore, a dynamic balance exists where validity is gained at the expense of reliability. Content validity is a subjective measure that cannot be evaluated statistically and is usually established by content experts. For a clinician-based outcome such as radiographic changes, the content experts may be a panel of physicians who together interpret the results. In patient-reported outcomes evaluating health-related quality of life, the patient may be the expert. Typically, content validity is best determined by directly examining the thoroughness of the instrument.

Criterion validity

Criterion validity examines how an outcome measure relates to an established gold standard in the same field. It is the most specific form of validity and the type most often considered in traditional medical research.

Construct validity

In contrast to content and criterion validity, construct validity is a more quantitative form of assessing the validity of an outcome instrument. A construct is an item or concept such as disease status, pain, or disability. Construct validity is evaluated by comparing the relationship between a construct within an instrument against a hypothesized similar construct within another instrument. For example, consider a functional instrument such as the disabilities of the shoulder arm and hand questionnaire (DASH) and a generic instrument such as the SF-36. In a patient with an upper extremity injury, one would expect that the functional scores of the DASH should correlate most with the functional scores of the SF-36 and expect less correlation between the functional scores of the DASH and the emotional measures of the SF-36.

2.2   Reliability

Reliability reflects the amount of random and systematic measurement error present within an instrument. Reliability of an outcome instrument is especially important when measuring the treatment effect of an intervention. If an outcome measure is not reliable, changes observed in the treatment group may not necessarily be attributed to the intervention, but rather, a problem inherent to the measuring instrument. Like validity, reliability is a dynamic property and is best assessed in terms of reproducibility and internal consistency (Fig 3-4).

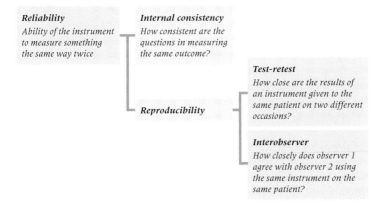

Reliability
Ability of the instrument to measure something the same way twice

Internal consistency
How consistent are the questions in measuring the same outcome?

Reproducibility

Test-retest
How close are the results of an instrument given to the same patient on two different occasions?

Interobserver
How closely does observer 1 agree with observer 2 using the same instrument on the same patient?

Fig 3-4 The components of reliability.

*Reliability is the ability of an outcome measure
to produce the same results with repeated assessment.*

Reproducibility

Reproducibility can be further subdivided into interobserver and test-retest reproducibility.

Interobserver reproducibility is the ability of a measure to produce the same results with repeated assessment by different observers rating the same experience. In other words, how closely does one observer agree with the interpretation of another observer using the same instrument? Interobserver reproducibility is described by kappa statistics.

Test-retest reproducibility, also known as intraobserver reproducibility, is the ability of a measure to produce the same results with repeated assessment by the same observer when no important dimension of health has changed. The test-retest reproducibility is estimated when administering the same instrument to the same patient on two different occasions. The result can be expressed in terms of a correlation coefficient. A highly reproducible instrument will have a high correlation coefficient between scores. These measurements may be complicated by a learning bias, where improvement in performance is attributed to completion of the instrument on a prior occasion. Understandably, correlation is dependent upon the duration of time elapsed between the two assessments.

Internal consistency

Testing internal consistency is appropriate when an instrument consists of several items forming a scale. The items or questions within the scale should be homogeneous, measuring the aspects of only one attribute. Most instruments employ several items to assess a single construct, based on the principle of measurement that several related observations typically produce a more reliable estimate than one. Thus, an instrument internally consistent is comprised of questions that correlate highly with one another and with the total score of items in the same scale.

2.3 Responsiveness

Responsiveness is assessed by comparing the outcome scores before and after an intervention and is calculated by the difference between the mean pre- and postoperative scores divided by the standard deviation of the preoperative score. It is possible for an instrument to be both valid and reliable but insensitive to change over time.

> *Responsiveness, also known as sensitivity to change,*
> *refers to the capacity of an instrument to detect clinically*
> *significant changes.*

Although of little significance when using dichotomous study end-points such as mortality or perioperative complications, this is extremely problematic when evaluating patient progress or the effects of a treatment over time. A measure that is not responsive may be of little clinical or research value even if valid and reliable.

> *Methodologically sound outcome instruments are valid,*
> *reliable, and responsive (*Fig 3-5*).*

> *Given the complexity of validating outcome tools,*
> *do not make modifications to accepted questionnaires,*
> *or try to develop your own instrument.*

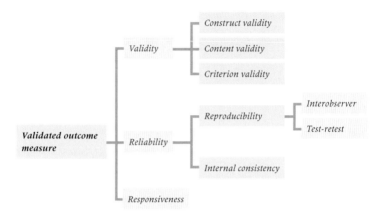

Fig 3-5   Summary of the components of a validated outcome instrument.

3   Clinical application of outcome instruments

An optimal health status measure has other desired properties in addition to appropriate content and sound methodology. The instrument should be easy to understand and complete by the patient while practical to administer and interpret by the clinician. Such instruments are said to be both patient friendly and clinician friendly. It is important that patients, who are already coping with a health problem, do not undergo any added stress from the instrument. Minimizing patient burden will maximize response rate and enhance data collection. Furthermore, a cost-effective, labor-friendly instrument reduces the resources required for data collection. The key concepts of patient and clinician friendliness are summarized in Table 3-1.

Patient friendliness

- *Can the instrument be completed in a relatively short period?*
- *Are the questions clear, concise, and easy to understand?*
- *Will patients be comfortable answering the questions?*

Clinician friendliness

- *Is the instrument completed by healthcare staff or self-administered?*
- *What is the staff effort and cost in administering, recording, and analyzing?*
- *How much time is required to train staff in administering the instrument?*

Table 3-1   The key concepts of patient and clinician friendliness.

The logistics of recording the outcome are another important factor in determining patient and clinician friendliness. Patients undergoing orthopaedic procedures often have mobility limitations and potential difficulty in attending regular follow-up visits required to document an outcome. Likewise, you rarely have the personnel available to complete frequent assessments. Therefore, outcomes requiring serial assessments, measurements, or imaging are for most purposes impractical. For instance, measuring the average time to union in order to assess the efficacy of a fixation technique is unreasonable because it would require the patient to undergo numerous x-rays.

Depending on the nature of the outcome, the route of administration may affect the validity of the results. For instance, health-related quality-of-life measures can be completed by personal interviews, mail-outs, telephone, and patient self-administration.

Your outcome instrument of choice needs to be clinician- and patient-friendly.

Repeated outcome assessments will enhance the informative value of your study, but are more difficult to accomplish.

The route of administration (ie, personal interview, mail-out) may influence both the rate and nature of response.

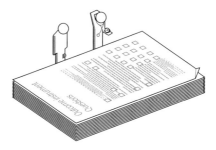

Fig 3-6   Huge outcome instrument may scare both patients and doctors, and may not suit clinical practice.

Each particular method has unique advantages and disadvantages to be considered. For example, consider the patient interview. You can clarify questions and ensure completion, thereby achieving a maximal response rate. Except patient interviews are costly and there is the potential for interviewer and reporting bias. Mailing-out on the other hand, is inexpensive and relatively unbiased, but response rates are generally low. The choice of the method to be used will depend largely on the research question, characteristics of the instrument, attributes of the patient population, and feasibility issues associated with cost and patient burden.

4   Limits and advantages of common outcome measures

Orthopaedic surgeons have a variety of options when considering outcomes for their studies. Since the interpretation of results and ultimately the inferences made within the study are dictated by the trial endpoints, investigators should select patient-important outcomes. For instance, one treatment protocol or intervention may be deemed superior to another based on a specific desired endpoint (eg, range of motion), but inferior based on another endpoint (eg, pain relief).

Therefore, it is possible for a well-designed study that clearly delineates superiority of one treatment over another to provide insufficient evidence or even be harmful if it fails to measure patient-important outcomes. In general, patient-important outcomes are changes that clinicians and patients regard as discernible and important, which have been detected with an intervention of known efficacy, or are related to well-established physiologic measures.

4.1   Clinician-based outcomes

Clinician-based outcome (CBO) measures such as joint range of motion, hardware positioning, gait abnormalities, and fracture union are often physiologic and assess the result of a healthcare intervention from the perspective of the clinician. They are often outputs rather than outcomes.

Objectivity is not determined by whether the clinician directly measures a parameter, but rather, is dependent on the reliability or reproducibility of a finding among patients and clinicians alike. Hence, many CBO measures are actually plagued with substantial variability. For example, interobserver agreement in determining motion of the spine or the extremities is often poor. It is also recognized that surrogate parameters (such as radiographic severity of osteoarthritis of the knee) correlate weakly with function and quality of life.

Many CBO measures have a tendency to use numerical scales to assign a point value to end results in orthopaedic trials. These numerical scales combine aspects of the clinical result (eg, range of motion, strength, radiographic changes) with the functional result (eg, pain, activity of daily living changes, occupational disabilities) to provide a final composite score.

The concern with such scales is that the weight (percentage of points on generally a 100-point scale) for each component is designated by orthopaedic specialists and not by the patients who have experienced the clinical injury or disease. Furthermore, the scores combine clinician-based data such as deformity and range of motion with patient symptoms within a single rating, despite the fact that these outcomes may vary independently.

Strenghts   CBO measures are not necessarily related to a patient's relief of symptoms, functional ability, or quality of life.

Limitations   CBO are available at the point of care and may also be derived from routine medical records.

4.2   Patient-reported outcomes

In contrast to CBO measures, patient-reported outcomes (PRO) are questionnaires or instruments completed by the patient rather than the health professional. They provide evidence and perspective distinct from that provided entirely by clinical assessment. This is especially important since multiple studies in other medical and surgical disciplines have shown that physicians and patients often significantly disagree about health status. This discrepancy is also present within the field of orthopaedics. For example, poor correlations exist between patient and surgeon outcome ratings of satisfaction following total knee arthroplasty. For proper evaluation of an intervention, the need to complement traditional CBO measures with patient-derived functional outcomes is now appreciated. The PRO instruments regularly used in outcome research measure general and disease-specific, health-related quality of life, patient symptoms, and functional status.

Strenghts   PRO measures what matters in healthcare and may be used for determening the value of a certain intervention.

Limitations   PRO is acceptable to individual thresholds of health perception. Especially after fractures and injuries, no baseline values are available.

4.3   Limiting bias in an outcome evaluation

The selection of an outcome should consider the susceptibility of that measure to bias and the potential for the use of bias-minimizing techniques.

> *Bias is a systematic tendency to produce a result*
> *that differs from the underlying truth.*

Biased outcome assessment, also known as ascertainment bias, compromises a study's validity and will ultimately lead to an underestimate or overestimate of the treatment effect. Clinicians can adhere to several methodological safeguards to limit such bias, including the use of validated outcome instruments.

Another useful practice is choosing measures that are as objective as possible, with the most extreme being dichotomous endpoints. A dichotomous outcome is one in which the result can equal only one of two possibilities. For example, a study participant is either dead or alive (mortality), or infection is either present or absent (postoperative complication) following surgery. Such yes or no outcomes are easy to record and are not subject to interpretation. Unfortunately, dichotomous outcomes may correlate poorly to a patient's own sense of well-being and have statistical limitations.

Bias-minimizing techniques include the blinded assessment and independent adjudication of outcomes. In other words, the outcome is determined by an independent healthcare provider or group of healthcare providers not otherwise involved in the study.

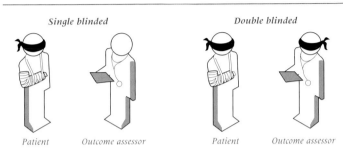

Fig 3-7 In a single blinded trial, the patient is not informed which of two or more interventions under investigation have been applied. This may impose ethical concerns and disturb the mutual trust of patients in doctors—it simply means "I know what you are receiving but I don't tell you". In a double blinded trial, neither patients nor doctors are aware of the assigned treatment. Obviously there cannot be a double-blinded trial of two different surgical interventions—however, it is still possible to have a blinded outcome assessor who had not been involved in the patient's treatment process.

As with treatment providers, outcome assessors carry their own expectations regarding the value of particular therapies relative to controls and are capable of consciously or unconsciously introducing bias. This is especially important in trials with outcomes that are subject to their determination. Unblinded assessors who are measuring or recording subjective outcomes such as clinical status, quality of life, or radiographic findings may provide preferential interpretations of marginal results thereby distorting the true treatment effect. By blinding, the outcome assessor is kept unaware of patient allocation, effectively reducing the potential for bias.

Double-blinded surgical trials are impossible, since this would mean blinding of the surgeon during the procedure. At best, surgical trials may be patient- and outcome-assessor blinded.

The more judgment involved in determining whether a patient has a target outcome, the more imperative blinding becomes. The study personnel assessing outcome can almost always be kept blinded, even if the patient and the operating surgeon cannot.

4.4 Typical dichotomous study endpoints

Dichotomous outcomes are unequivocal trial endpoints such as mortality, reoperation and the presence of infection. These endpoints have only two possibilities, where the study participant's outcome must be one or the other and cannot be both. Continuous endpoints, in contrast, consist of data measured on a continuum or scale (range of motion or time to union). Typical dichotomous and continuous endpoints in orthopaedic trials are listed in Table 3-2.

Study endpoints in orthopaedic trials

Dichotomous measures	Continuous measures
• Complications	• Functional/clinical score
• Reoperation	• Radiographic results/scores
• Implant failure	• Mobility/ambulatory status
• Nonunion/union	• Range of motion (degrees)
• Pain	• Time to union
• Infection	
• Segmental collapse	
• Avascular necrosis	

Table 3-2 Typical dichotomous and continuous endpoints in orthopaedic trials.

Dichotomous endpoints are popular in orthopaedic research being advantages in several aspects. Ease of statistical analysis with the use of risk or odds ratios and more importantly, ease of interpretation make these outcomes attractive to investigators. In clinical practice, this translates into improved understanding of study results by decision makers. For example, the impact of an intervention that reduces mortality or the incidence of infection is easy to appreciate. In outcome assessment, dichotomous measures are objective and therefore not subject to misinterpretation. This effectively reduces the introduction of ascertainment bias (bias outcome assessment).

From a logistics perspective, the recording of dichotomous measures is clinician friendly. The resources required to record and analyze an endpoint such as mortality are not as substantial as an endpoint requiring numerous technical measurements over multiple assessments (eg, range of motion, functional status).

For analysis and presentation purposes, investigators have the tendency to dichotomize outcomes. That is, converting an outcome previously measured on a continuous scale (eg, range of motion) into two separate values (limited or unlimited) around a clinical threshold. The drawback with such simplifications is that information about the size of the treatment effect may be lost (absolute immobilization versus moderate limitations in range of motion). Additionally, the appropriate clinical threshold where the outcome is segregated is subjective and difficult to determine.

The difficulty with many dichotomous endpoints is that the measured outcomes are typically infrequent and, therefore, differences between treatment modalities are very small. The risk, for example, of pulmonary embolism as a complication following total hip arthroplasty is estimated at approximately 1%. The smaller the clinical difference the investigator wishes to detect, the larger the sample size required to power the study. It is often not feasible to conduct large trials of surgical therapies in orthopaedics. Therefore, trials of small sample size with dichotomous endpoints are at risk of lacking sufficient statistical power to draw definitive conclusions. In orthopaedic literature, small studies with continuous outcomes have significantly greater study power than those that report dichotomous outcomes.

> *Dichotomous outcomes are easier for investigators to manage and understand, but have statistical limitations.*

Strenghts of dichotomous outcomes such as surgical revision, yes/no, or death/alive are objectivity and easy interpretability. For this reason, dichotomous endpoints are often named hard endpoints. There is no doubt whether the event of interest has occurred or not; it cannot be misclassified, and you cannot turn back the clock. For clinicians, dichotomous endpoints are easier to communicate to patients, and studies providing a yes or no answer are more likely to change clinical practice.

Limitations   are imposed by rather small treatment effects (specifically in trauma and orthopaedics) and the need for large sample sizes. As we have currently reached the ceiling with many surgical interventions, it is difficult, if not impossible, to demonstrate a marked improvement in event rates. In addition, dichotomous endpoints often do not reflect patient needs and opinions.

5   Functional scores

Functional status measures an individual's ability to perform the normal daily activities necessary to meet basic needs, fulfill usual roles, and maintain health and well-being. Two related concepts, functional capacity and functional performance, characterize a patient's functional status. Functional capacity represents an individual's maximum ability to perform daily activities in physical, psychological, and social domains. Functional performance refers to the activities people actually carry out during the course of their daily lives.

Example   *In the case of a patient with severe arthritis of the hand, maximal grip strength measures physical functional capacity, while a self-report of tasks completed at home measures functional performance.*

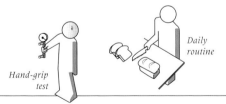

Daily routine

Hand-grip test

In musculoskeletal disorders, the distinction between functional status and health-related quality of life measures is particularly difficult. A continuum exists between instruments that focus on physical function and those that also include a broader range of health dimensions, such as emotional and social functioning. With respect to functional status, functional scores are by far the most common measures in terms of numbers available. In some conditions, they are too numerous, often complicating comparisons of results across different scales. Two validated measures of functional status in the orthopaedic literature are the Western Ontario and McMaster Universities osteoarthritis index (WOMAC) and the DASH scores.

For a more comprehensive review of functional score measures refer to the AO Handbook—Musculoskeletal Outcomes Measures and Instruments, 2nd expanded edition (Suk et al).

6 Health-related quality of life

The World Health Organization (WHO) defines health as "a state of complete physical, mental, and social well-being, and not merely the absence of disease". Therefore, a measure attempting to quantify a patient's health must capture each of the aspects of well-being simultaneously and summarize them in a single metric. The instruments accomplishing this task are referred to in orthopaedic literature as health-related quality of life (HRQOL) measures. These measures differ from those that document quality of life in that they do not include personal values, socioeconomic status, environment, opportunity, and social network. Rather, HRQOL focus generally on the aspects of quality of life directly affected by a health condition. In patients with musculoskeletal disorders, HRQOL relates generally to physical function, role functioning, and symptoms.

Advances in orthopaedic surgical procedures have shifted the assessment of outcome from the success or failure of a procedure towards changes in patient functional status and quality of life. Traditional medical measures such as blood tests and imaging studies often do not provide definitive answers about whether a treatment is useful or successful from patient perspective and may even poorly correlate with a patient's own feelings of well-being. HRQOL measures facilitate clinicians' understanding of what patients believe has been gained or lost as a result of an intervention. Therefore, patient-derived functional outcome data should be a major driver of treatment protocol for the musculoskeletal disorders.

Health-related quality of life instruments are organized into generic and disease-specific measures (Fig 3-8).

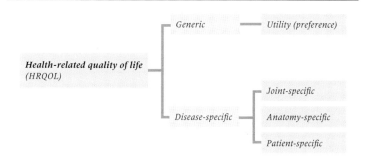

Fig 3-8 Different categories of health-related quality of life measures.

6.1   Generic measures

A generic health-related quality of life instrument quantifies a patient's perception of his or her overall health status. This includes physical symptoms, function, and emotional dimensions of health. The sickness impact profile (SIP), the Nottingham health profile (NHP), the SF-36, and the EuroQol questionnaire (EQ-5D) are examples of generic instruments. Since they measure overall health rather than a specific condition, generic instruments are useful for comparing health status across different diseases and severities, interventions, and even across different cultures. Heart disease, diabetes, obesity, and other comorbid health issues are incorporated along with the orthopaedic problem into the measurement. Due to their wide range of clinical applications, however, generic instruments are prone to abuse. Clinicians, often overwhelmed by number and variety of outcome measures available, may default to the use of a validated generic instrument when a potentially more appropriate or sensitive measure is in fact available. Generic instruments regularly lack the sensitivity to detect small but clinically important changes, specifically with orthopaedic disorders.

Utility or preference measures are a unique form of generic instrument that measure health status by placing a patient's health on a continuum from perfect health or well-being to death. Through placement on a continuum with anchors of death and full health, preference measurement provides a means to compare alternative interventions, patient populations and diseases. Cost-utility analysis can be used to measure the cost-effectiveness of competing interventions in which the cost of an intervention is related to the number of quality-adjusted life years (QALYs) gained.

One QALY equates 1 year of life in perfect health. Likewise, 0.5 QALY equate 6 months of life in perfect health, or 1 year of life with a 50% reduction in health-related quality of life. QALYs are among the most important indicators of effectiveness for health policy decisions.

Individual patient preferences may be queried by techniques such as the time trade-off (TTO); weighing time in current health state versus a shorter time in complete health, and the standard gamble (SG); weighing trading current health state for improved health state that also comes with risk of death. They are used to obtain a utility value.

6.2 Disease-specific measures

Disease-specific measures of health-related quality of life are tailored to inquire about physical, mental, and social aspects of health specific to injury (eg, fracture), disease (eg, osteoarthritis), anatomical area (eg, knee), or a population of interest (eg, athletes). Specific measures of single concepts or conditions are the most numerous outcome instruments within the health status field. The popularity of these measures primarily arose from the need of clinical trials and practitioners for accurate scales responsive to clinical changes that occur over time. In contrast to their generic counterparts, disease-specific instruments are better able to detect smaller or important changes that occur over time in the particular disease studied. This specificity has also been shown to contribute to a more responsive measure.

7   Practical issues of selecting appropriate outcome measures

The relative benefits and limitations of the various types of scores and health-related quality of life measures are dependent on their intended use and the type of information sought. These measures may be used to evaluate outcomes at a point in time, to predict future outcomes or events and to measure important clinical changes over time. If you are looking for information with regard to a single patient, a disease-specific instrument may be appropriate since generic measures rarely have the precision to be useful at an individual level.

If evaluating a program or group of patients, you may add a generic measure to allow for comparison of the group with population norms, or across different disorders.

Utility measures are often of use to health economists requiring a preference rating for economic analysis.

Generally, the recommended approach has been to include both a generic and disease-specific outcome measure to ensure adequate assessment. In reality, many granting agencies and ethic approval boards insist that a generic instrument be included in the design of proposed clinical trials.

8   Summary

- Choosing appropriate outcome measures is vital for the success of your project. The primary outcome of your study will determine both the sample size and the clinical impact of your results.

- Surrogate measures (such as laboratory or radiographic findings) are outputs and may not necessarily correlate with outcomes (ie, function, patient satisfaction, quality of life, etc).

- In a clinical trial, always consider at least one patient-reported outcome (ie, a generic or disease-specific health questionnaire) as primary or secondary endpoint.

- Choose outcome measures with known validity, reliability and responsiveness. Do not try to "modify" established instruments, or dissipate your energies with developing your own scale or score.

4 The perfect database

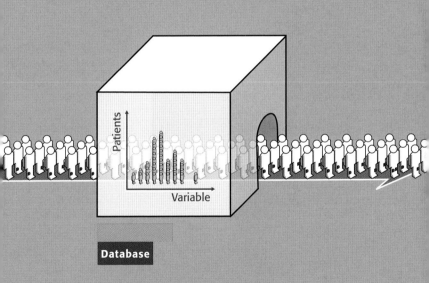

Variable

Patients

Database

4 The perfect database

4   The perfect database

1   Introduction

A database is a structured collection of information that is stored in a computer system and organized in such a way that it can be quickly accessed and retrieved. The database is the treasure chest of your scientific project and may contain confidential, patient-related information, and other highly sensitive records.

You need to plan data collection diligently and strategically at the very beginning of your study, always keeping in mind that any information collected must be processed and stored in some way. With newest generation hardware and software there is almost no limit in the volume of data you can store. Nevertheless, there is a limit to the amount of data that can be practically dealt with. It is impossible to keep track of, let us say, more than 100 items with 200 patients enrolled in a clinical study. Discipline and restrict yourself. Don't let your enthusiasm overwhelm your project. If you try to know everything about your patients, procedures, treatments, outcomes, your enthusiasm will quickly fade, and be replaced by frustration. It is impossible to answer all questions in one single study, so don't even try.

> *It is better to have a limited but complete dataset than a million incomplete entries.*
>
> *If you fill in nonsensical information you will receive meaningless output ("garbage in, garbage out").*

Since data must be processed electronically, it is important to use a code understood by computer software. This often requires using numerical rather than alphanumerical language. However, we must also be capable of easily retranslating numbers into clinically meaningful information. Thus, defining your list of items is always a trade-off between simplification (for the sake of smooth data storage and processing) and complexity (to ease clinical interpretation).

Database files on a computer can be created in many ways. Programs suitable for producing a database range from common word processing software to specialized database systems. The choice of a specific program depends mainly on the complexity of the data to be stored in the database and on the functionality required for entering and managing data. Though database creation and management is not the primary intended function of spreadsheet programs (such as Microsoft Excel®), it has become very popular among researchers for this purpose. Spreadsheet packages support many tasks involved in creating and maintaining a database without requiring highly specialized technical expertise. For that reason, the following account on the perfect database will focus on the use of spreadsheet programs. However, most hints and recommendations could also apply to other programs. It is noteworthy that many statistical packages have similar data entry and editing procedures. Even genuine database systems like Microsoft Access™ provide data tables in a format very similar to a generic spreadsheet.

2   The basic database

A database presents in the form of a table consisting of rows and columns. In each column a specific type of information is stored. All information belonging to a given case is collated in one row of the table. The rows of a table in a database are called "records", the columns are called "fields" or "variables".

To illustrate this typical row-column format, individual patient data in Table 1-1 of chapter 1 "About numbers" were entered into a spreadsheet table (Table 4-1). Assume we consider a cohort study that compares two different femoral nails (1 = entered via the trochanteric tip; 0 = entered via the trochanteric fossa) for intramedullary fixation of femoral shaft fractures. It can be seen that all information from Table 1-1 was transferred literally into the spreadsheet table, including headings in the first row describing the content of each column below. Interestingly, this spreadsheet table is already an (almost) perfect database.

Columns—fields/variables

Rows—records

ID	pseudo	male	age	tip_nail	dur_surg	n_blood
1	TANUR877	1	18	1	91	0
2	MOLUT504	0	25	1	49	0
3	METUT536	1	49	1	68	1
4	BOMUK480	1	58	0	71	2
5	MUSUR955	1	71	0	63	5
6	BIBUT318	0	50	1	55	3
7	BEMEL434	0	40	0	109	0
8	NOBUT546	1	31	0	45	0
9	BUMUK835	1	69	1	60	0
10	SUBON450	1	54	1	67	1
11	RABAB061	1	58	0	90	1
12	LARUT055	1	82	1	84	2
13	SUTUT761	1	19	0	56	4
14	RUBUS526	0	47	1	79	0
15	ROMUS580	1	31	1	64	0
16	BANON356	0	59	0	102	0
17	NUNUT119	1	67	0	61	3
18	LAKUK515	1	69	1	53	2
19	MIBEL627	1	73	1	50	1
20	SEBUR182	0	84	0	4 7	1

Table 4-1   Results from a hypothetic randomized trial of femoral nails entered via
the trochanteric fossa or the trochanteric tip.

A few points should be noted in order to make a table a nearly perfect database.

First, a rectangular row-column format is required, and a unique heading must be assigned to each column.

> *It is important that each column has its own unique heading because statistical software packages accessing the database use this information to distinguish between the fields or variables.*

Column headings should be descriptive but brief, eg:
- "male" is better than "column_3"
- "n_blood" is better than "number_packed_red_ blood_units_surgery"

In general, headings should consist of no more than eight characters and numbers. Short names are often much easier to deal with in statistical packages. If more information is necessary in the printed results, most statistical programs allow for extended labeling to describe the content of a variable in more detail. Column headings should begin with a character followed by a mixture of characters and numbers (eg, "date", "date1", "date1postop").

Special symbols like $, #, %, -, or & and embedded blanks should be avoided. The only exception is the underscore ("_") which is accepted by most statistical programs. As some statistical packages are case sensitive and others are not, it is better not to rely on upper/lower case to distinguish variable names.

Secondly, for each patient a unique patient ID should be entered. This is not mandatory but makes life much easier when the content of the database needs to be checked against the original data, when single cases or groups of cases must be selected for specific purposes, or when data on the same patients from other sources are merged into the existing database. You may have noticed that, in addition to the ID, each patient was assigned a pseudonym (indicated by "pseudo").

Regulatory authorities, international rules for the conduct of trials, and laws of data safety discourage the use of patient indicators (eg, the first two letters of the given and the surname). Individual patients must not be traceable from the information recorded in your database. For this reason, the patient's age, but not birthday should be recorded. A pseudonym, such as the randomly generated alphanumerical code (five letters, three numbers) used in the above example, must be created for each subject in your database. A linkage file that allows for identifying an individual patient by his or her pseudonym must be stored separately from the database, and access should be restricted to few people involved in the project.

Thirdly, all entries in the records contain precisely the information described in the column headings (gender of the patient entered consistently as "male" or "female"; age; type of nail used, ie, tip or trochanteric entry; duration of surgery; and units of packed red blood as numerical data). In this example; male and female gender, and the type of nail was coded as 0 or 1. If the variable of interest has only two expressions (such as male or female) that are mutually exclusive, it is better to use a true binary code (1=yes, 0=no) rather than "male/female", "yes/no", or "1/2". The binary code is natural in this setting, and is recognized by statistical software.

Question marks or other information added to an entry or comments in separated columns generally cause serious problems.

Finally, if there is some reason to use character data (in our example "male" and "female"), it is essential to follow exactly the same spelling throughout (and not "male" and "Male"). Otherwise, data analysis will report as many categories as there are different ways of spelling.

3   Dos and don'ts in the use of spreadsheets for data entry

3.1   General format

Data should always be arranged in rectangular format. Each row of the table shows the information collected for one case (avoid empty rows); each column comprises information about one specific characteristic of the cases.

> *Avoid empty rows by entering data on consecutive rows from the top to the bottom of the spreadsheet.*

If the data set comprises several groups of patients, the data for each group should be placed on the spreadsheet one after the other and a column should be included indicating to which group the cases belong.

> *All the data should be on one spreadsheet.*

No other information than just the plain data (and column headings) should be given into the spreadsheet. Calculations of means or other statistics or a comment make a spreadsheet very difficult to use for input to statistical packages.

> *Refrain from using special text formats (boldface, italics), colors, shading or frames to avoid complications when data are accessed from other programs.*

3.2   Entries

Each cell in the data table should contain precisely the relevant data—nothing else. In a column containing numeric data, never use "?" alone or in addition to an entry to indicate something is still unclear, nor use "grade 2/3 open fracture" if it is still to be determined whether the entry is "2" or "3".

It will be necessary to find consensus in this situation, either by discussing the individual case with colleagues, by having an independent review, or by clearly indicating that there is an equivocal or indeterminate result. If this happens rarely, it will probably not affect your study findings. If it frequently occurs, you must find a solution to avoid bias by so-called misclassification.

You may consider:
- Introducing an extra category like "unclear/borderline/transitional classification"
- Performing best-case and worst-case analyses, with your variable either classified as 2 or 3

If information is missing, a special code for missing data should be created. For numeric data, any value that does not occur as a valid entry may be used to flag missing data. Codes of 9, 99, 999, … are traditionally used for this purpose.

Information consisting of several items of information should be disaggregated as much as possible. For example, the information that a patient received 500 mg of aspirin three times daily should not be entered in a column "medication" simply as "ASS 3 × 500mg". Instead, three columns containing each of the relevant items should be used (Table 4-2).

a	medication_type	medication_times	medication_dose_mg
	Aspirin	3	500

b	AO_fx_type	AO_group	AO_subgroup
	B	2	2

Table 4-2a–b
a   It is much easier to combine different items of information into a composite than to decompose a complex entry like "ASS 3 × 500 mg".
b   Similarly, a Müller AO Cassification of Fractures in Long Bones B2.2 fracture should be classified using three columns.

4   A spreadsheet package or more advanced database programs?

Spreadsheet packages are very useful tools for data entry and storage and a good choice in many circumstances. However, their capacity to deal with large and complex data sets is limited and they provide only few options for generating data entry forms, checking data upon entry, or the automatic skipping of fields conditional on previously entered information. If complex data sets have to be managed, eg, longitudinal patient data with a variable number of visits during a study, or if advanced data entry procedures are required, the use of a specialized database program, such as Microsoft Access™ or FileMaker®Pro software, should be considered.

From a data entry point of view, the main advantages of specialized database programs are the availability of user-generated data entry forms and data checks upon entry. Fig 4-1 shows a data entry form for the patient data of our initial example (this form was generated using Microsoft Access™). At first glance, this may appear to be just a cosmetic version of a row for data entry in a spreadsheet. However, the sophisticated validation rules and consistency checks that can be incorporated when using such a form are hidden. Correct data entry can be guaranteed by entry checks. Users may be guided in a way that only numbers are accepted in numerical fields. In the field "gender" you can guide with "male" or "female", "yes" and "no", or "0" and "1" . A unique numerical identifier can be provided for "patient-ID", and only values greater than or equal to 0 can be ascertained in the blood packs field. Moreover, fields can be defined as "must enter", plausibility checks can be implemented and skip patterns conditional on information in certain fields can be imposed.

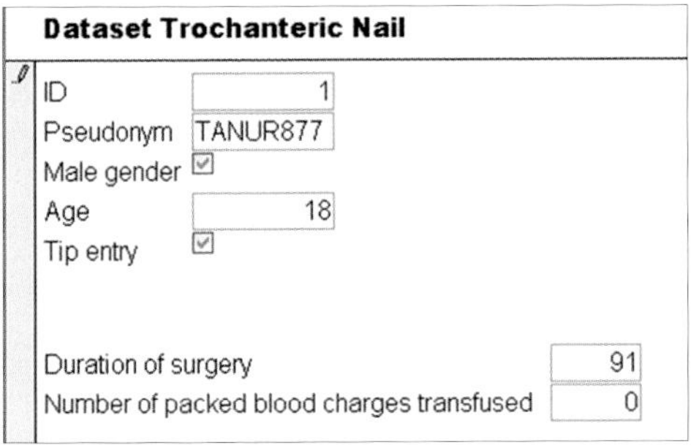

Dataset Trochanteric Nail

ID	1
Pseudonym	TANUR877
Male gender	☑
Age	18
Tip entry	☑

Duration of surgery	91
Number of packed blood charges transfused	0

Fig 4-1   Microsoft Access™ data entry mask.

Against the background of these advantages of specialized database programs, their primary disadvantage is that, because of their sophistication, they require a certain degree of technical knowledge and expertise. While experienced users may quickly create a database and entry forms within a database program and include appropriate validation rules, the occasional user may need to invest more time for database programming than for setting up an "almost perfect" spreadsheet for data entry. For this reason many users of spreadsheet packages continue to use this method for data entry and data management. If the simple rules given in the previous section are followed, spreadsheets can be a good alternative to more sophisticated and more complex database systems.

5 Some ways to ensure data quality

5.1 Validation rules

Imposing validation rules at the time of data entry is a powerful tool for preventing errors. With range checks, checks of permitted numerical and character input, errors can be detected and corrected immediately when they occur. If the data entry system does not provide these checks simultaneously, they can be applied as a second step after data entry has been completed. Minimum and maximum values in a data column as a range check for numerical values can easily be determined even in a spreadsheet environment. Frequency tables of numerical or character data belong to the core functions of all statistical packages and are very useful for detecting data entry errors. As these second-line checks are performed mostly after completion of data entry they are more time consuming than real-time validation. If an error is detected, the original data forms usually have to be consulted.

5.2 Consistency checks

Data are inconsistent if the information in one variable is incompatible with the information in another. A date of surgery prior to the date of hospitalization, prostate cancer as co-morbidity in a female patient, or a period of 5 days sick-leave in an unemployed patient are typical examples of such inconsistencies. While such inconsistencies are easily recognized once they have been identified, they are difficult to eradicate because a large number of logically impossible combinations of data may exist. Researchers should invest appropriate time to define as many potential inconsistencies as possible. With a clear and comprehensive list of such inconsistencies a data analyst can easily check if any of these actually occur in the database, for example by calculating the time elapsed between the day of hospital admission and the day of surgery, tabulating comorbidity separately for male and female patients, or by comparing the days of sick-leave for patients with different occupational status.

5.3   Double data entry

No validation rule or consistency check will help in case of erroneous entries, for example, if the duration of surgery was 86 minutes but the digits 6 and 8 were entered in reverse on a computer keyboard. Double data entry is the only strategy to avoid or at least to minimize the likelihood of this type of error. This very effective method for quality control should be used whenever possible. It is best to enter all data twice; however, if resources are restricted, double data entry for a subset of cases and/or a limited number of variables may provide an estimate of the reliability of the data.

6 Summary

- The database is the treasure chest of your scientific project.

- Plan the number of variables and their description wisely, and take care of it. Since it may contain patient-related data, it must be stored and secured. Ensure that no patient-related information is accessible to anybody not involved in the planning and conduct of your study (ie, use pseudonyms and a separate linking file).

- To be processed by statistical software, a rectangular row-column format is required, and a unique heading must be assigned to each column. All variables must be precisely defined. A code book may be a good idea.

- Headings should be descriptive, bot not exceed 10 alpha-numeric characters. Avoid symbols except "_".

- Never make more than one enry in one cell.

- Missing data should be flagged by a number not used in your dataset (eg, 999). Use "1" and "0" to indicate "yes" or "no".

5 How to analyze your data

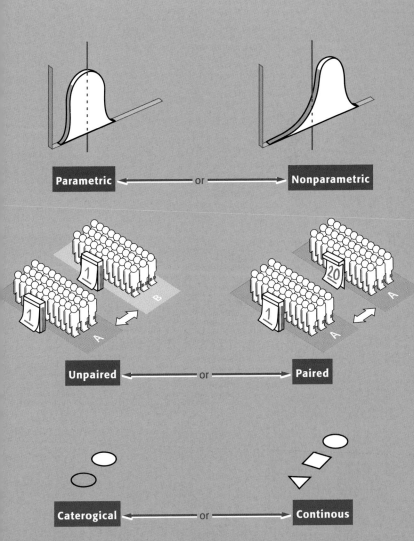

Parametric ←———— or ————→ Nonparametric

Unpaired ←———— or ————→ Paired

Caterogical ←———— or ————→ Continous

5 How to analyze your data

5   How to analyze your data

1   Statistical tests: the basics

Statistical methods for data analysis have a long history, and biostatistics has emerged as an own, prospering field of research. Powerful statistical software has been developed that allows for thorough calculations on large datasets that would be impossible to be performed manually. Some of the available methods are complex and difficult to apply, while others can easily and successfully be employed by researchers without a strong statistical background. Luckily, the most common statistical analysis methods in biomedical research belong to the latter category. Don't let statistical software seduce you to do computations you cannot understand—if in doubt keep it simple, since you are responsible for the interpretation of the results.

The most common statistical approach in biomedical research is the analysis of differences that may exist between two or more groups of patients: Is postoperative pain intensity lower in patients after minimally invasive versus conventional total hip replacement? Are women more likely than men to develop anxiety disorder after severe injury? Are extraarticular type A fractures associated with better functional prognosis than intraarticular type B or complex type C fractures? You may argue that, if the difference is large enough, statistical tests are dispensable—and you are right. However, in case of moderate or small differences, the key question is, whether the observed effect has occurred simply by chance. This is what statistical tests are made for.

> *Statistical tests are tools that distinguish between results compatible with chance, and those that no longer can be explained by chance.*

Also, all statistical tests share the same principle—they compare the observed results with an expected value, based on your dataset, and come up with a so-called test statistic. This statistic is compared to a tabulated value derived from the underlying distribution. If the statistic is higher than a certain critical or threshold value, the difference between observed and expected results is no longer a matter of chance. All of these different steps of computation and comparison are nowadays made by statistical software.

> *In research practice, it is important to know which tests should be used for which kind of data, and why a particular test may or may not apply to your research question.*

2   How to choose the appropriate test

The good news is that the choice of the appropriate statistical method for comparing groups is often straightforward. In most cases, the suitable method depends only on two criteria—the number of groups (two versus more than two) and the data type (binary, categorical, ordinal, continuous) involved in the comparison. Only when group differences with respect to a continuous variable are analyzed a third aspect, namely the choice between "parametric" and "nonparametric" methods, plays a role. When the data can be assumed to follow a normal (Gaussian) distribution in each group, a parametric method is appropriate. Nonparametric, or so-called distribution-free methods can be used in those cases where this assumption does not apply (in fact, they can be used for all types of data, but this is a little too simple).

Many popular statistical tests for analyzing differences between groups, such as the t-test, analysis of variance (ANOVA), or the chi-square (_2) test can be integrated in a framework of analysis methods based on our three decision criteria—number of groups, data type, and assumption of normal distribution. An overview of some common methods for analyzing group differences based on these criteria is shown in Table 5-1.

		Data type			
		Binary or categorical	Ordinal	Continuous	
Number of groups				Normal distribution assumed	Normal distribution not assumed
2	Descriptive statistic significance test	Proportion chi-square test	Median Mann-Whitney U test	Mean value t-test*)	Mean value Mann-Whitney U test**)
3+	Descriptive statistic significance test	Proportion chi-square test	Median Kruskal-Wallis H test	Mean value ANOVA (F-test)	Mean value Kruskal-Wallis H test

Table 5-1   Appropriate methods for statistical analysis of differences between groups.

*) sometimes referred to as "Student's t-test".

**) also known as "Wilcoxon rank sum test".

When only two groups will be compared a simple example can illustrate the use of this table:

Example   *Suppose a fictitious randomized clinical trial of conservative versus operative treatment of fractures of the scaphoid.*

Only patients who are working at the time of the injury are enrolled in the study. Duration of sick leave represents the primary endpoint. A total number of 60 patients are randomized to receive either conservative (short-arm cast) or operative treatment (Herbert screw fixation).

The occurence of complications such as malunion, nerve compression, or wound infection (yes/no) represents the primary endpoint. Secondary endpoints comprise ratings of pain and discomfort at 6 months after the injury (no pain or discomfort, pain or discomfort at strenuous exercise, pain or discomfort at minor exercise, continuously). Also, patients are followed-up and the time until return to work will be recorded.

*The onset of a complication is binary, or dichotomous—
a patient will or will not encounter an adverse event.
Hence, we would compare proportions (or percentages) and
use the chi-square test.*

*Pain and discomfort is an ordinal variable comprising
only three categories. Here we would compare the medians and
use the Mann-Whitney U test.*

*Duration of sick leave is a continuous variable (it may,
in theory, range from zero to hundreds of days).
The difference between the two treatment groups can
be analyzed by comparing the mean values of this variable.
If the data are normally distributed, the t-test would be
the appropriate statistical test. Otherwise, the nonparametric
Mann-Whitney U test would be the relevant method.*

3 Binary or categorical data

The primary endpoint in our example, occurrence of complications, was measured in two categories (0: no complication, 1: one or more complications). This binary variable can easily be analyzed using proportions or percentages (percentages are proportions multiplied by 100). In Table 5-2, the fictitious results for this binary variable are shown.

	Treatment group		Chi-square test
	Conservative (N = 30)	Operative (N = 30)	P value
Percentage with complications	10.0	20.0	0.278

Table 5-2   Statistical comparison of occurrence of complications in patients after conservative and operative treatment.

It turns out that the incidence of complications in the conservative group (10 %) was lower than in the group with operative treatment (20 %). While this difference of 10 % in favor of the conservative group may be relevant from a clinical point of view—depending on the kind and severity of complications—a statistical test should indicate whether this difference can have been produced by chance. The null hypothesis in this case is that the percentage of complications is the same in both groups and equal to the marginal percentage of complications when both groups are combined (ie, 15 %). The chi-square test (denoted by the Greek letter "chi" to the power of 2: $\_2$) can be used to test this null hypothesis.

Results of this test are also included in Table 5-3. Because the P value is greater than the prespecified significance level of 0.05 we conclude that the null hypothesis, the proportion of complications is equal in both groups, can not be rejected. Hence, it is decided that the observed difference was produced by chance.

> *The chi-square test can be used in situations where binary data for just two groups are being compared.*
> *In this case the chi-square test is equivalent to a significance test of the odds ratio (OR) or the risk ratio (RR). When testing the odds ratio or the risk ratio the null hypothesis is that OR = 1 and RR = 1, respectively.*
>
> *The chi-square test can also be used in situations where binary data for more than two groups are being compared. The previous comments about difficulties with pairwise comparisons using nonparametric methods apply here also.*

Application of the chi-square test requires the sample size to be "large enough". A rule of thumb states that this condition is met when none of the expected frequencies calculated according to the null hypothesis is smaller than 5.
If this is not the case it is recommended that either a corrected version of the chi-square value (applying the "Yates' correction") or a method known as "Fisher's exact test" is used. Most statistical programs provide results for all three tests, P values for the chi-square test, the corrected chi-square test, and for Fisher's exact test.

4   Ordinal data

In our example, pain and discomfort was assessed using a discrete variable with a small number of categories (A: no pain or discomfort, B: pain or discomfort at strenuous exercise, C: pain or discomfort at minor exercise or continuously). With only three levels the ratings of pain and discomfort are not really a continuous variable. It must further be assumed that the distances between adjacent response categories are not equal. However, the categories are clearly ordered. For analyzing the results for this endpoint, the Mann-Whitney U test is appropriate (see Table 5-1).

When using the U test, instead of comparing values of the arithmetic mean, we rank order the entire data set and compare the mean ranks obtained for the two groups. The distribution of the pain and discomfort ratings and respective results from the Mann-Whitney U test are displayed in Fig 5-1.

The marked differences in the pain and discomfort ratings between the two groups are in favor of the operative treatment. This difference in the rank ordered data is also statistically significant ($P = .033$), demonstrating that not only the sick leave data but also the patient reported outcomes show differences in the same direction.

For comparisons of more than two groups the nonparametric equivalent to the F-test used in the analysis of variance is the Kruskal-Wallis H test. Again, a significant result of this test only indicates that the data are not compatible with the null hypothesis of no differences between groups. The test result will not tell us which of the groups differ significantly from each other. In contrast to the parametric analysis of variance, where a number of methods for pairwise comparisons are available which avoid overadjustment for multiple testing, nonparametric tests of pairwise differences mostly rely on Bonferroni correction or a modified, less conservative method, the Bonferroni-Holm correction.

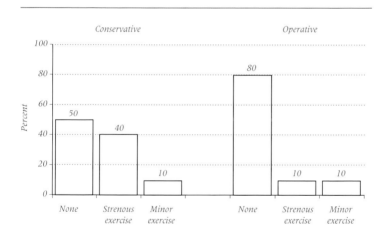

Fig 5-1   Pain and discomfort ratings of patients after conservative and operative treatment.

5 Group comparisons involving continuous data

Continuous data, such as age or time until return to work, can take any value within a specified range of minimum and maximum value. Some variables are not strictly continuous in this sense but can only take a certain number of distinct values. The Injury Severity Score (ISS) or a numerical rating scale for pain intensity with 11 categories from 0 (no pain) to 10 (worst imaginable pain) are examples of such data. If the number of distinct values is large enough there is little reason not to treat them as if they were "truly" continuous.

For the primary endpoint in our example, duration of sick leave after the injury (measured in weeks), we accepted that this is a continuous variable. In Fig 5-2 the fictitious results of the study are shown.

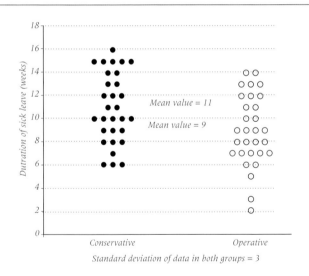

Fig 5-2   Duration of sick leave for patients under conservative and operative treatment.

The average number of weeks until return to work was 11 weeks in the conservative group and 9 weeks in the surgical group. The difference of 2 weeks between the two regimens does not seem to be very impressive. Yet, given the standard deviation of 3, this difference is two thirds of the standard deviation.

Having observed this difference of 2 weeks of sick leave between the treatment groups, the investigator will usually be interested in whether this difference is "statistically significant". To answer the question whether a difference between groups is statistically significant is equivalent to answering the question whether this difference can be explained merely by chance. For testing statistical significance, we (hypothetically) assume that both treatments are equally effective with respect to duration of sick leave and that the observed difference simply occurred by chance. This is the "null hypothesis". Then, based on the value of a relevant test statistic, the probability of obtaining the observed difference, or one more extreme, under this assumption is computed. This probability is called the P value. If the P value is less than or equal to a prespecified probability level, the so-called significance level, the result is said to be "statistically significant"—the occurrence of the observed difference just by chance would be so unlikely that we reject the hypothesis that both treatments are in fact equally effective. The significance level most often used in statistical tests is 0.05 or 5%. This value is no natural constant, but simply a convention (see also chapter 2 "Errors and uncertainty").

> *A significance level of 5% is only a convention, but reasonable and accepted in the scientific community.*

Depending on the circumstances, smaller (eg, 0.01, 0.001) or larger (eg, 0.10) significance levels can be chosen. Even though the particular choice of the significance level is a bit arbitrary it is very important that it is defined in advance before the test is conducted and not post hoc after the P value has already been obtained.

As can be seen from Fig 5-1, the data for the primary endpoint are not completely normal. The distribution of the variable in the conservative group is more compressed than a normally distributed variable would be and the operative group has two cases with a very short duration of sick leave. Many statistical methods exist for assessing whether empirical data are consistent with a normal distribution. However, this is rarely needed—a pragmatic way is to graph your data first to gain an impression of the underlying distribution.

> *Do descriptive and graphical analyses first before proceeding with statistical testing.*

Our data seem to be sufficiently normal so that a parametric test for statistical significance of the difference between the two groups is justified. According to Table 5-1, the appropriate statistical test for comparison of mean values in two groups is the t-test. Alternatively, if we don't trust that the data come from normal distributions, the nonparametric companion of the t-test, the nonparametric Mann-Whitney U test can be used. Results of both analysis methods are presented in Table 5-3.

	Treatment group		t-test (parametric)	U test (nonparametric)
	Conservative (N = 30)	Operative (N = 30)	P value	P value
Mean value	11.0	9.1	0.016	0.024
Standard deviation	3.0	3.0		

Table 5-3   Statistical comparison of duration of sick leave in patients after conservative and operative treatment.

With the usual significance level of 0.05 both the parametric t-test and the nonparametric U test indicate that the difference is too large to be attributable to chance alone. We therefore reject the null hypothesis of equal outcomes in both treatment arms.

A respective manuscript summarizing the results of the study could read in the "Methods" and "Results" sections:

Example

> *Methods: ... Differences between the two groups were tested by the t-test. The results were considered to be significant if P < .05 ...*

> *Results: ... The patients treated by surgery were on sick leave for an average of 9 ± 3 weeks compared with 11 ± 3 weeks in the patients treated conservatively (P = .016) ...*

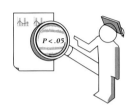

We tacitly employed a so called "two-sided test". This means that we expected that significant differences could occur in both directions, favoring either conservative or operative treatment. If a real difference can be assumed to occur only in one direction a "one-sided test" would have been the correct method. However, one-sided tests are rarely appropriate in medical research.

The standard t-test requires the standard deviations in both groups to be equal—an assumption which can also be statistically tested. If this assumption is violated an alternative t-test is available. Almost every statistical program will provide the user with the results of the standard and the alternative t-test.

The printed output of statistical test results often show a magic quantity: the "degrees of freedom". This is simply a technical number that is a function of either the number of cases in the sample and the number of groups or, when contingency tables are analyzed, of the number of rows and columns in that contingency table.

6   Comparison of more than two groups

Consider now a similar experiment in which two surgical treatments (say, a titanium Herbert screw and a new bioresorbable screw) have been included in the study protocol in addition to the conservative treatment arm. Now the comparison involves three instead of two groups. According to the overview in Table 5-1, analysis of variance (ANOVA) and the associated F-test would be the relevant statistical analysis method. The null hypothesis to be tested with the F-test is that the mean values of all three groups are equal. If the statistical test gives a significant result this only tells us that this null hypothesis is not consistent with the data. Sometimes this will be exactly what we wanted to know. Yet, we would still not know which of the differences—between the titanium and resorbable screw, between the titanium screw and conservative treatment, or between the resorbable screw and conservative treatment—are unlikely to occur when in fact no differences exist (Fig 5-3).

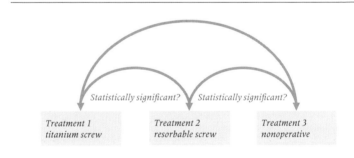

Fig 5-3   Pairwise comparisons of three groups.

Generally, if k groups are involved, a total number of $\frac{(k-1) \times k}{2}$ pairwise comparisons are possible—in our example with three groups the number of comparisons is $\frac{(3-1) \times 3}{2} = 3$. To answer the question which of the differences are statistically significant it may be tempting just to conduct t-tests for all pairwise differences. Such multiple t-tests are usually a bad choice. The reason is that multiple testing is associated with a "true" significance level that is larger than the nominal value of, say, 0.05. In this situation, a null hypothesis of no difference will be rejected even if the probability that the difference occurred by chance is larger than the prespecified significance level. Another choice, the so-called Bonferroni correction by dividing the nominal alpha level by the number of comparisons $(0.05/3 = 0.017)$ and rejecting the null hypothesis if the P value is less than or equal to the corrected significance level avoids the problems of the inflation of the significance level. However, this method is likely to overadjust the significance level and hence to miss existing differences. Statisticians call this property of the Bonferroni correction "conservative".

> *As a rule of thumb, the Bonferroni method is better than ignoring the implications of multiple testing.*

If Bonferroni-corrected results are statistically significant, the researcher is on the safe side because the difference is at least "as significant" as or even "more significant" than the nominal alpha level. More complicated situations may require the application of specific multiple-comparison methods which avoid overadjustment.

7   Analysis of paired data and other extensions

Paired data arise when the observations are related in some natural way: an endpoint is measured before and after an intervention, presence of a certain disease is assessed in pairs of twins, cases and controls are matched according to relevant characteristics. It would be a mistake to use the methods described above for analyzing differences between groups with such paired data. Ignoring the process that generates the paired data (repeated measurements, matching) will almost always produce wrong results of statistical tests. Fortunately, for all examples described here, methods that account for paired data are available. When only two variables are paired, the paired t-test (continuous data), Wilcoxon signed-rank test (ordinal data), or McNemar test (binary data) can be used. With more than two related observations per case (measurement of outcome before and after treatment and 6 months later, for example), repeated measurements ANOVA (continuous data), the Friedman test (ordinal data) and the Bowker test (categorical data) are appropriate.

Even though the methods for statistical data analysis presented in this chapter cover a wide range of approaches to answer specific questions of scientific interest, a researcher can be confronted with situations in which these methods are not sufficient. A common challenge in data analysis arises when the effects of more than one factor on outcome variables have to be taken into account simultaneously. Then, multivariable methods like linear or logistic regression are required. Application of multivariable methods is not necessarily much more difficult than using the methods included in this chapter, yet, they require—as can be expected with advanced techniques—a deeper understanding of the underlying statistical principles and at least some experience in their application. It is always a wise decision to seek advice from a statistical expert if you have any doubts about appropriateness of a particular statistical method.

---

8   Summary

- The results from statistical tests indicate whether an observation may have been produced simply by chance.

- Statistical tests compare the difference between expected and observed values.

- The choice of the appropriate test depends on the quality of data (binary, categorial, continuous), the underlying distribution (symmetric versus shewed), and the dependency of groups (paired versus unpaired).

- All statistical problems that go beyond need qualified assistance.

---

6 Present your data

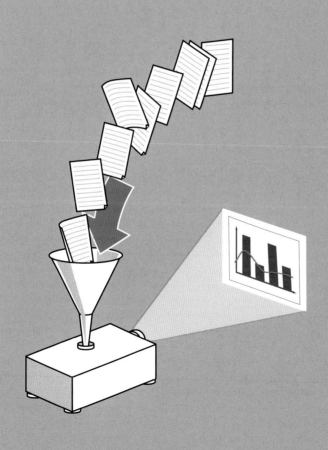

6   Present your data

6   Present your data

1   We are visual people

"A picture is worth a thousand words"—everyone knows this famous proverb.

Figures and charts are the most influential vehicles for distributing scientific information. They may affect the acceptance or rejection of a manuscript, and the reception of study results by the scientific community. Unfortunately, they have also become popular tools to cheat both health care professionals and consumers as well.

Apart from formal statistical analyses, a graph gives a distinct impression on the effect size, the center and distribution of values, and outliers. As physicians, specifically surgeons, we are visual people, and often grasp the essentials from a clinical study more effectively by graphical than by numerical presentation.

Mastering the most common types of charts is a key to successful data interpretation, be it the first analysis of your own study results, or the critical appraisal of a widely cited paper that is on its way to affecting your daily practice. Regardless of the setting, forget everything you learned in your art classes about colors, light, and canvas. Do not attempt lush paintings when designing your graphs, and be alert where others have: they may have simply tried to paint over weaknesses in their source data.

2 Scientific figures are simple but clear

The most comprehensive and clear figures are artistically boring. However, it was the famous architect Louis Sullivan who, in the late 19th century, coined the phrase "form follows function." We will respect this principle in this chapter, adhering to the following three golden rules to achieve graphical excellence:

> *Aim for the highest possible data density*
> *(that is, the amount of information provided per graph area).*
>
> *Lower your ink-to-data ratio*
> *(ie, do not use unnecessary shading, 3-D, grid lines, and other elements often called "chartjunk").*
>
> *Label axes clearly and unequivocally.*

A figure tells a story, and byplay seriously distracts readers from the key message. Please keep in mind: the selective use of color may greatly enhance information flow and highlight the key message in a slide presentation, but has little, if any, meaning in a scientific manuscript (other than in photographic images such as histological sections). Since most journals do not publish color figures due to high printing costs, it makes almost no sense to submit them for peer review. The graphical features of commercial software like Microsoft Excel® or advanced statistical packages are seductive, and researchers may feel that color jazzes up their figures or makes them more impressive.

> *If it needs color to draw attention to a figure, it is probably useless.*

If information is new and important, a black-and-white line drawing will be sufficient and self-explanatory. Thus, learn how to express information with few graphical elements.

The researcher's essential graphical tool box should contain histograms, bar charts (always with measures of error), box-and-whiskers plots, scatter plots, and forest plots. We will show how to design and use these.

3   Your graphical masterplan and toolbox

You made it—you completed a randomized trial of a new locking plate versus a conventional T-plate for open reduction and internal fixation of an A3 distal radial fracture according to the Müller AO Classification of Fractures in Long Bones. After 1 year of follow-up, the disability of the arm, shoulder, and hand (DASH) score in both groups comes up as shown in Table 6-1 (keep in mind that lower DASH scores mean better function).

Patient	Disability of the arm, shoulder, and hand (DASH score)	
	Locking plate	T-plate
1	12	6
2	15	16
3	5	8
4	4	11
5	9	6
6	8	8
7	12	6
8	13	18
9	4	13
10	1	17
11	1	20
12	14	19
13	15	17
14	13	4
15	5	21
16	2	2
17	8	9
18	12	14
19	7	10
20	10	12

Table 6-1   Results from a hypothetic randomized trial of locking plate versus T-plates for internal fixation of distal radial fractures.

DASH scores in the locking plate and T-plate group average 8.5 ± 4.6 and 12.0 ± 5.8. How can you illustrate this difference, for yourself, your co-workers, and the scientific audience?

4 Bar charts

Your research assistant makes a first proposal, as depicted in Fig 6-1. You remember the three golden rules of graphical excellence? Did your research assistant meet any of them?

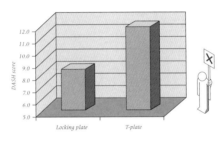

Fig 6-1 A busy bar chart depicting the mean values from Table 6–1.
- Shading and 3-D has no information content
- Low data density
- Tiny fonts
- Labeling incorrect and incomplete

The figure is filled with uninformative chart junk (shading, 3-D) and has a very low data density (in fact, it contains only two values—the mean DASH score in both groups). But can you trace the meaning easily from the figure? No, since the y-axis is not labeled. You also realize that the figure suggests a quite large difference between study groups, because the y-axis stretches from 5–12, not from 0–12. Finally, note the ratio between the figure size and the font size. Tiny fonts further impede abstracting of information from the figure.

Now throw this figure in the dustbin; start again, but systematically. Remember the aim of figures. They are vehicles for transmitting condensed information and must be fully comprehended even at a glance. Do not let your figure confuse the readers' eyes. Feed the audience, let the information rush directly into their brains. This guarantees retention and sustainability of your results in the scientific community.

The bar chart remains the most common way of graphical data presentation. It is easy to understand, and you may have already created bar charts that resembled those displayed in Fig 6-2. Note that Fig 6-2 contains the same information as Fig 6-1, but with a much higher data density, correct axis scale, and appropriate labeling.

However, with a little extra effort, you can produce bar charts of ultimate informative content. We invite you to become a perfect bar-charter.

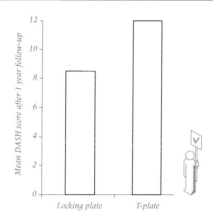

Fig 6-2   Bar chart depicting the mean values from Table 6-1 but:
• Higher data density
• Correct axis scale
• Appropriate labeling

5   Error bars

5.1   Clinical relevance

Do not only picture mean values or percentages, but also use a format that shows distributions and outliers. It clearly makes a difference whether your mean value of 8.5 was derived from a range of 4–10, or 0–25. The perfect graph shows both the clinical relevance and statistical significance of study findings. In case of symmetrically distributed data (like ranges of motion, functional scores, and quality of life measurements), use the standard error of the mean (SEM) or the standard deviation (SD). Both are appropriate but indicate your choice unequivocally, either at the y-axis or in the figure legend.

The meaning of error bars must clearly be specified.

Remember the SEM is always tighter than the SD (the SEM results from dividing the SD by the square-root of the sample size). Since this suggests a higher precision (Fig 6-3), authors sometimes omit to indicate that their error bars are SEM, not SD. If in doubt, the SD is the better option. Most readers will expect error bars to represent SD, not SEM. Also be sure that error bars in both groups expand in both directions. Imagine you had obtained DASH scores in your distal radius fracture trial after 3, 6, and 12 months (Fig 6-4). By contrasting the upper range of one group to the lower range of the other group, one gains the optical illusion of a large difference between study groups.

Error bars must be two-tailed, since patients may always experience results better or worse than the average population.

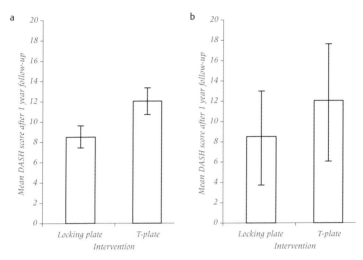

Fig 6-3a–b   Always specify the meaning of error bars.
a   SEM.
b   SD.

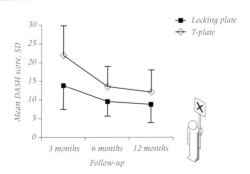

Fig 6-4   One-tailed error bars skew the data because of optical enlargement of the differences.

5.2 Statistical significance

Beside clinical relevance, the statistical significance of your findings can best be expressed by incorporating a 95% confidence interval (95% CI) into your chart (Fig 6-5a). As a rule of thumb, it is unlikely that observed differences have been produced by chance, if the 95% CI of mean values (and proportions) do not overlap. Conversely, overlapping 95% CI mean that the observed differences are still compatible with chance (or a P value $> .05$, if this was chosen as the level of significance).

In addition to the 95% CI of means or proportions of either group, you may also present the difference in means or proportions together with the 95% CI and the exact P value (Fig 6-5a). The entire information on the primary endpoint of the trial can be traced from a single figure:

After 1 year of follow-up, locking plates were associated with a slight advantage in function, as indicated by a mean difference of 3.4 points

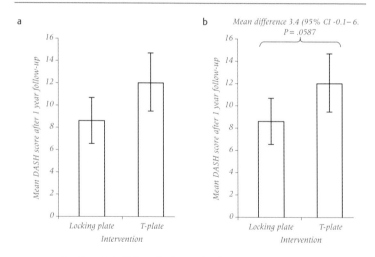

Fig 6-5a–b   Provide statistical information in your chart by 95% confidence intervals.

in the DASH score (Fig 6-5b). This observation was, however, still compatible with chance since the 95% overlap and the 95% CI of means includes the null.

6   Box-and-whiskers plots

Box-and-whiskers plots (or box plots), originally proposed by Tukey, have become an important alternative to bar charts when displaying continuous data. In contrast to bar charts, they contain detailed information about the center and distribution of data in your sample. The anatomy of a box plot is displayed in Fig 6-6, using the example of a case series of proximal humeral fractures. The box plot shows the difference in DASH ratings between the baseline assessment and after three months of follow-up with conservative treatment.

By convention:
- The box always contains the interquartile range (the "tenderloin" of your data set).
- The bottom line of the box represents the 25% percentile (in this graph, 25% of all differences are lower than zero. 25% of all patients had already achieved their previous shoulder function).
- The transverse line represents the median, or 50% percentile. The median cuts your data set into half (see also chapter 1 "About numbers", Fig 1–6). In our example, 50% of all patients had less than 5 points difference between baseline and follow-up DASH scores, the other 50% had more than 5 points difference.
- The upper margin of the box equals the 75% percentile. 75% of all patients had differences below 18 points.
- The remaining 25% had differences of 18 points and more compared to their preinjury status.
- The whiskers represent the range of values outside the box length.

- All values below and above the whiskers are individual extreme observations, so called outliers, and are represented by circles or dots.
- Sometimes, apart from the median, the mean value is indicated by a square or a diamond in the box.

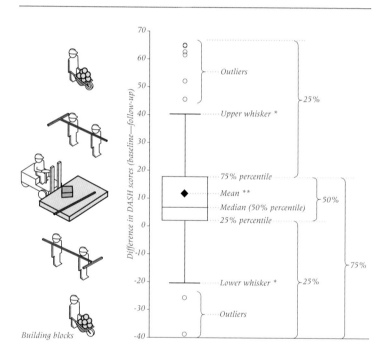

Fig 6-6   Anatomy of the box-and-whiskers plot.

*) The definition of whiskers vary (in this example, they include values that are within 1.5 times the box height).

**) Mean values are not always provided in the box, but nicely demonstrate whether the underlying distribution is skewed.

In the original work, whiskers represented the range of values that were within 1.5 times of the box length.

This definition is, however, not straightforward, and recent descriptions suggest displaying the 10% and 90%, 5% and 95% percentile, or even the minimum and maximum instead. Refer to the instructions of your software package for the individual default setting. If you consider using another whisker meaning than the default, specify your choice in the figure legend.

Do not think about the interpretation of whiskers too long—just accept it. It's one of many conventions and recommendations in statistics.

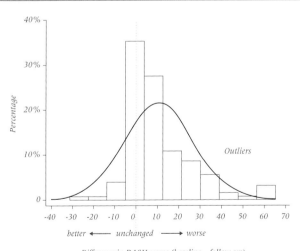

Difference in DASH scores (baseline—follow-up)

Fig 6-7   Note that important values (median, interquartile range) are difficult to be traced from this type of figure.

The corresponding histogram is shown in Fig 6-7, and highlights the enormous data density of the box plot. The histogram is still a commonly used method for data presentation. Although it fully illustrates the distribution of data, it is difficult to trace important values (median, interquartile range) from this type of figure.

Comparison of findings by box plots is quick and easy (Fig 6-8). Again, box plots display a range of discrete or continuous data. They cannot be used if your primary outcome is binary (ie, yes or no, 0 or 1, healed or failed, and others).

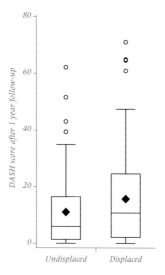

Fig 6-8   Comparison of subgroups by box plots—DASH scores after 1-year follow-up in patients with undisplaced and displaced fractures.

Almost all commercial statistical software packages (like SPSS®, SAS®, STATA®, and others) offer sophisticated box plot options. Although Microsoft Excel® has comfortable graphical features, it currently does not allow for producing box plots simply by a mouse click. However, many committed Excel® users have found extremely clever ways to produce box plots with the available graphical tools in just a few steps.

Strenghts   With very few lines and less space than a histogram, the box plot illustrates the center and largest portion of data (the central 50%), and indicates whether the underlying distribution is skewed (in the example, the median is about 5, while some outlier values between 45 and 65 drag the peak of the normal curve towards a mean of 10).

Limitations   It needs some time to become familiar with the meaning of the different lines in a box plot. The box plot may obscure important information (see Fig 6-15). The interpretation of the whiskers varies considerably in the scientific literature, and also depends on the software package used for statistical analysis.

7   Scatter plots and regression lines

Sometimes you may be interested in displaying the association between two continuous measures. For example, the difference in DASH scores (as in Fig 6-6 and Fig 6-7) may depend on the patients' age.

Plotting the difference in DASH against age may result in an association as depicted in Fig 6-9. But what is wrong with this figure? Of course, the regression line, since it is not backed-up by observations made in patients younger than 65. It is not justified to assume that, although there may be a slight linear association between age and difference in DASH scores in elderly patients, this is also true for younger subjects (that had not been included in the cohort).

Regression lines must not exceed the range of observations.

When presenting the results from regression analysis, include 95% CI as well to illustrate the uncertainty of predictions when your independent variable of interest (eg, age) reaches the extremes of your dataset. Also, a study with a smaller sample size may, on average, come to conclusions similar to those of a large investigation, but with less precision (Fig 6-10).

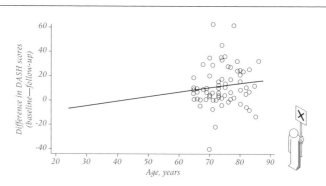

Fig 6-9   Unjustified extension of the regression line to an area without observations.

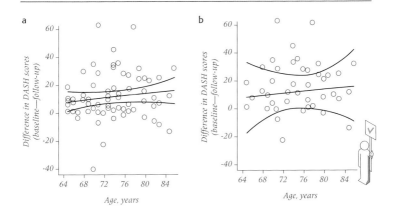

Fig 6-10a–b
a Widening of the 95% CI at the edges of the dataset.
b Similar slope of the regression in a comparable but smaller study with wider confidence intervals.

Strenghts   The scatter plot takes advantage of the full range of data and visualizes associations between variables very well.

Limitations   The scatter plot does not indicate a causal relationship between "x" and "y" and is space-consuming.

8 Forest plots

Finally, your results may show interesting diversity among subgroups of patients. Of course, you can create multiple bar charts or box plots, or provide a table. There is, however, an elegant and emerging option to graphically display differences in outcomes between subgroups. You may use meta-analyses (eg, Cochrane reviews) for evidence-based decision making in your daily practice, and thus be familiar with forest plots.

> *Forest plots allow for viewing the results from all subgroup analyses at once (*Fig 6-11).

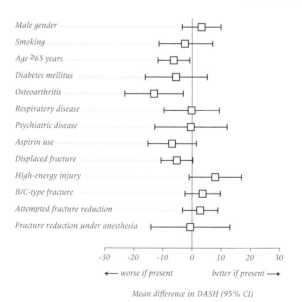

Fig 6-11   A forest plot to illustrate the results from subgroups analyses.

The tendency of mean values away from the null suggests trends (eg, worse outcomes in patients with displaced fractures compared to those with undisplaced fractures). By studying whether the 95% CI includes the null value, you can also distinguish statistically significant from statistically nonsignificant associations at the $P < .05$ level (in case of patients ≥ 65 years or those with osteoarthritis). Always keep in mind that the results from subgroup analyses are nonconfirmative.

> *Results from soubgroups only suggest trends and generate hypotheses for future studies.*

We have already stressed that the more you test, the more likely there will be a false-positive finding simply by chance. The famous 5% threshold can be misleading—one in twenty trials will result in a positive result.

Strenghts   The forrest plot format is now accepted by most journals as a graphic of choice for illustrating the results from subgroup and metaanalysis.

Limitations   The forest plot format is sometimes difficult to understand, and needs additional numerical information or a comprehensive legend.

9   Your personal way to graphical excellence

Pie charts belong to the graph types with the lowest data density. The best advice is to completely avoid them in a scientific presentation or manuscript. Fig 6-11 sketches an example. Although it fully illustrates the distribution of data, important values (median, interquartile range) are difficult to be traced from this type of figure, published in the report of a randomized trial of hook pins versus screws for the internal fixation of cervical hip fractures (Fig 6-12a). The authors aimed to show the time interval between admission and surgery. Because the interval was separated into seven categories, multiple colors were needed to build a chart which still does not allow for reading the individual proportions. The presented graph clearly missed its target, and could have been replaced by a histogram (Fig 6-12b).

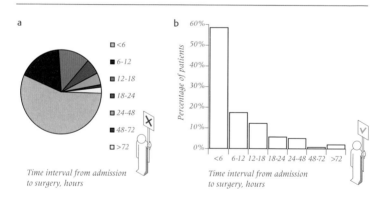

Fig 6-12a–b
a   This pie chart was intended to show the proportion of patients scheduled to surgery
    at different time intervals. However, percentages cannot be traced from the diagram.
b   The histogram is efficient, catchy, and does not need color.

Stacked bar charts may be confusing if they contain more than two or three categories, as shown in Fig 6-13. The best probable alternative to this space-consuming, uninformative graph would be a table (Table 6-2).

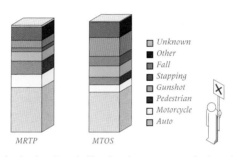

MRTP   MTOS

Fig 6-13   Low data density of a 3-D stacked bar chart that compares mechanisms of injury of patients enrolled in the modal rural trauma project (MRTP) and the major trauma outcome study (MTOS).

Cause of injury	MRTP	MTOS
	n = 266	n = 80544
Unknown	5 (1.7%)	81 (0.1%)
Other	35 (13.2%)	11921 (14.8%)
Fall	16 (6.0%)	13290 (16.5%)
Stabbing	10 (3.8%)	7652 (9.5%)
Gunshot	22 (8.1%)	8054 (10.0%)
Pedestrian	32 (12.0%)	6041 (7.5%)
Motorcycle	32 (12.0%)	5558 (6.9%)
Motorcar	106 (39.8%)	27949 (34.7%)

Table 6-2   Data table corresponding to Fig 6-13.

Schriger and Cooper stressed the need for distinguishing between unpaired and paired observations. Fig 6-14a shows the pre- and post-operative ranges of motion (ROMs) in elbow joints of 14 patients undergoing surgical resection of heterotopic ossifications. Again, the figure contains much chartjunk. Box plots would have pictured the gain in ROM simpler and clearer than the original figure (Fig 6-14b).

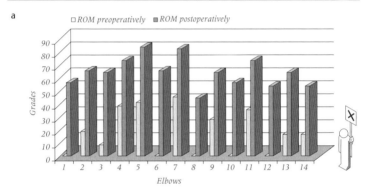

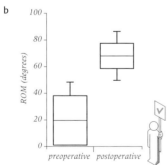

Fig 6-14a–b   Handling of paired data.
a   Data presentation with plenty of information.
b   Box-and-whiskers plots of preoperative and postoperative ranges of motion (ROMs) provide equivalent information with a much higher data density index.

However, in a box plot summery measures (eg, mean, median) may obscure the worsening of function in single patients. In case of small sample sizes (ie, around 20–25 subjects), one-way plots may reveal both overall trends and individual patients' courses (Fig 6-15).

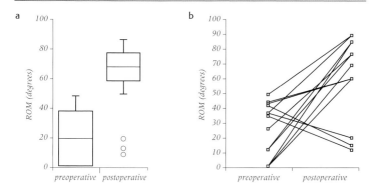

Fig 6-15a–b   Handling of paired data—if individual information is of high interest.
a   The box-and-whiskers may obscure individual data, eg, obscure the worsening of function in three patients, and moderate effects in another two.
b   A one-way plot provides the full scope of information (that is, the individual effect of surgical resection in all patients).

If you can handle bar charts, histograms, box plots, scatter plots and regression lines, and forest plots properly, you will be able to present most scientific data relevant to orthopaedics and trauma in a highly professional manner.

Graphs that go far beyond (eg, survival curves, receiver operating characteristics) should remain in the hands of your statistical advisor.

10   Summary

- Strategically plan the partitioning of study results into figures, tables, and text.

- Data related to the primary hypothesis may be elegantly presented in a first-order graph like a bar chart, box plot, or scatter plot, together with appropriate measures of error and distribution.

- Whenever possible, 95% confidence intervals should be added to allow the reader to assess both relevance and significance of the findings.

- Data from subgroup or stratified analyses, or those related to secondary hypotheses can be presented graphically (eg, box plots for different strata), or tabulated. Further results considered noteworthy (eg, conflicting with current evidence, or otherwise generating hypothesis) may be explained in the text.

- Figures must replace but not repeat written text. As a rule of thumb, a figure is needed if a written passage is far more complex to comprehend than an illustration (eg, "After 3, 6 and 12 months of follow-up, radiographic healing was noted in 45/104 (43%), 90/104 (87%), and 98/104 (94%) fractures in the experimental group. In the control group, these numbers were 24/100 (24%), 82/100 (82%), and 96/100 (96%).")

7 Glossary

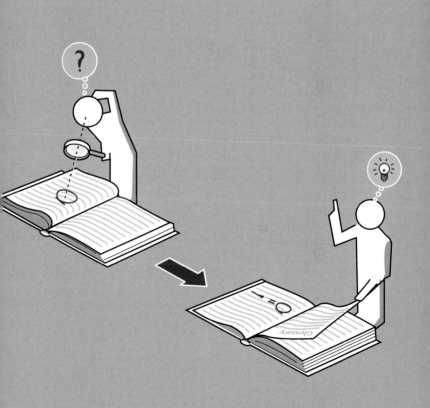

7 Glossary

association   Two variables are associated if some of the variability of one can explain some of the variability of the other. Do not confuse with "causality". Two variables may be associated simply by chance (eg, the size of miniskirts and stock exchange prices) (see pages 8, 9, 11, 19, 31, 39, 126, 127, 129).

bias   Bias is a systematic (often unrecognized) deviation of measurements from the truth. If you want to measure the appropriate length of a locking screw, but scale of your gauge is incorrect, you will always choose screws that either do not grip the second cortex or protrude into the soft tissue (see pages 21, 34–36, 38, 39, 62, 66, 69–71, 87).

blinding   In a blinded experiment, the subjects do not know whether they are in the treatment group or the control group. In order to have a blind experiment with human subjects, it is usually necessary to administer a placebo to the control group. It is obviously impossible to have a double blinded trial of two surgical interventions—you could, however, conduct a patient—and investigator blinded trial (see page 70).

categorical variable   A variable with a usually small range of possible expressions without a hierarchical order or prognostic implications (eg, blood group). If the variable has a scale format with higher values indicating a stronger impact on the outcome of interest (eg, severity of fracture comminution from B1 to C3), it is called ordinal.

causation   Two variables are causally related if a change in the value of one is necessary to induce a change in the other. It is the primary goal of any research project in biomedicine to explain the degree of causality between an exposure (eg, a treatment intervention or risk factor) and the observed outcome. Consequently, there is a vast body of philosophical and theoretical work on causation, including certain rules that mean a causal relationship is very likely (eg, plausibility, strength of the effect, reproducibility, and many more).

chi-square test   The most common test procedure for evaluating statistical differences in binary or categorical outcomes (ie, those that can be put in cross-tables) (see pages 96–100).

cohort study   A longitudinal study in which subjects are exposed to different risk factors or treatments, and are followed-up to determine whether there is a difference in outcomes (see pages 19–23, 82).

confidence interval   The confidence interval is the prespecified range of values that the observed average is still compatible with. Typically, a 95% confidence interval (CI) is provided. This means that if you repeated your study 100 times, the observed average would be within the confidence limits at least 95 times (see pages 50–52, 120, 127, 134).

confounding   Confounding is present if the differences in outcomes between groups are apparently caused by an exposure such as a certain treatment, but in fact have another cause associated with the exposure. Confounding is mainly a problem in observational studies. For example, obesity may be linked to higher complication rates after orthopaedic procedures, whereas the true cause of the complications is diabetes associated with obesity.

continuous variable   A quantitative variable is continuous if, in theory, it can reach infinite values (although lower and upper margins are usually within biological limits). Examples include temperature, height, age, and many others. In both clinical and methodological practice, discrete variables (such as those from functional scores) are handled as continuous as well (see pages 10, 96, 98, 100, 102).

correlation   A measure of distinct, linear, or nonlinear association between two (ordered) lists (slightly stronger than association). Similar to association, two variables can be strongly correlated without having any causal relationship (see pages 59, 61, 62, 68).

cross-sectional study   In a cross-sectional study, individuals are compared to others at the same time. The case-control study is the archetype of cross-sectional studies. Individuals are sampled with and without a certain condition of interest, and exposure variables are retrospectively evaluated. Cross-sectional studies allow for a glimpse on the population, and are conducted if longitudinal assessment is impossible (see pages 21–23).

deviation   Deviation expresses the difference between a datum and some reference value, typically the mean of the data. Probably best recognized is the standard deviation (SD) that illustrates how widely data spread around the sample mean. As a rule of thumb, the mean plus one, two, and three SDs cover 68%, 95%, and 99% of all observations in the data set (see pages 48–52, 63, 102–105, 118).

distribution   Distributions explain how values show up and scatter in a certain data space. The well-known normal distribution represents a bell-shaped curve, but there are multiple other distributions your statistician will consider when selecting the most appropriate analysis strategy (see pages 14–16, 28, 32, 33, 43, 45, 47, 48, 51, 52, 95–97, 100, 104, 109, 113, 118, 121, 122, 124, 125, 130, 134).

event   Events occur or do not occur—there is nothing in between. There are beneficial events (like solid union) and adverse events (like infections), that may represent the primary or secondary outcomes of your study. Sometimes, it takes more time for an event to occur than you are capable of following up patients. In this situation of uncertainty, observations may be censored (see pages 16–19, 22–28, 31, 38, 47, 55, 72, 77, 98).

hypothesis   The hypothesis is the formalized expression of your idea, containing both qualitative (what, where, and when) and quantitative (which size or degree) components. Posing a clear, unequivocal, and answerable research hypothesis is the very first step when designing a clinical study. It always should be issued in the format "we hypothesize that x is equal to or n times better than y in treating z", or similar (see pages 31, 32, 38, 99–101, 103, 104, 106, 107, 134).

hypothesis testing   Biomedical statistics follow the principle of falsification. When you set out to demonstrate advantage of x over y, your null hypothesis should read "x is equal to y" (literally meaning there is an exact null difference between x and y). Your study aims at producing data that allow for rejecting the null hypothesis, and allowing for accepting the alternative hypothesis that there is a difference between x and y.

interquartile range (IQR)   The interquartile range of a list of numbers is the upper quartile (or 75% percentile) minus the lower quartile (or 25% percentile). Thus, the IQR contains the central 50% of all your observations. It should be provided together with the median (see pages 13, 123, 124, 130).

linear association   Two variables are linearly associated if a change in one is associated with a proportional change in the other (see page 126).

longitudinal study   A study in which individuals are followed over time. They may be compared with themselves at different times, to determine, for example, the long-term effect of an intervention on some measured variable. At different time intervals, there may also be a comparison to a control group (see cohort study). Longitudinal studies provide much more conclusive evidence about time-dependent effects and causal relationships than cross-sectional studies. However, they need many more resources.

mean (or arithmetic mean)   The sum of a list of numbers divided by the number of numbers (see pages 10, 14, 15, 16, 28, 32, 33, 37, 43, 45, 48–51, 63, 86, 97, 98, 100, 102, 104, 106, 116–120, 122, 125, 128, 129, 133).

median   The "middle value" of a list of values—this cuts your dataset into half. Exactly 50% of all values are above or below the median. The median is robust against outliers and the preferred index if data are skewed (see pages 13–15, 28, 97, 98, 121–125, 130, 133).

number needed to treat (NNT)   The NNT describes how many patients need to be treated by one intervention compared to another to either prevent one undesired event (eg, a nonunion), or to induce one beneficial event (eg, solid union). It represents the inverse of the risk difference (RD) (see pages 26–28).

odds ratio   The odds ratio (OR) is the typical measure in cross-sectional studies. It expresses the relative likelihood of an individual who has a certain condition or disease of having been exposed to a certain risk factor or treatment. In contrast to risk ratios or relative risks (RR) it trades-off "winners" against "losers", rather than "winners" against all participants of a study. The rarer the event, and the higher the sample size, the more the OR approaches the RR (see pages 18, 23, 28, 71, 99).

outlier   An outlier is an observation that is many standard deviations from the mean. It is sometimes seducing to discard outliers, but this is neither justified or sound, nor helpful. An outlier may indicate an interesting finding that needs to be explored in detail, and discarding outliers may lead to underestimation of the true variability of the measurement process (see pages 14, 32, 113, 118, 122, 123, 125).

***P* value**   The *P* value is probably the least understood, but most frequently used statistical index in biomedicine. Discussing its background and meaning would probably inflate this glossary to the size of an encyclopedia. For consumers: The *P* value is the probability that certain information derived from a study is compatible with chance. The lower the *P* value the lower the probability that an observation has been caused by chance alone. The (nearly) correct interpretation is: *P* is the probability of observing data similar to, or more extreme than the observations made, given the null-hypothesis is true. The "magical" 5% threshold established in the medical sciences is purely a convention, not a natural constant. It reflects the pragmatic assumption that if only one in twenty experiments turn out positively by chance, there must be some underlying causal relationship between the exposure and outcome of interest (see pages 11, 39, 40, 98–100, 103, 104, 107, 120).

power The power is the probability of demonstrating a difference (in fact, of coming up with a statistically significant result) given there is a difference between an experimental and the control intervention. Of course, if you believe in the effect of a novel treatment rather than the standard of care, you are interested in showing this in a clinical study. The power is calculated as 1-type II error, and driven by both the size of the effect, and the sample size of your study. The larger the demonstrated effect or sample size, the larger the chance you can show it in your study. This also means that the lower the effect, the larger the target sample size must be, and vice versa. By the way—it makes no sense to do so-called "post-hoc" power analyses, you have to do this a priori. If a study turns out negative—fate. Never argue "if we had included this or that number of patients, we would have come up with positive results". You have to have consent on the relevant effect size in advance, not later. Also—if there are statistically significant differences, it is not necessary to calculate the power of your study anyway (see pages 41, 72, 99).

quartiles There are three quartiles. The first or lower quartile of a list of numbers contains 1/4 (or 25%) of the numbers in the list that are no larger than it. Likewise, 3/4 (or 75%) of the numbers in the list are no smaller than the third or upper quartile. The second quartile (or 50%) is the median (see pages 13, 28).

randomized controlled trial (RCT) The RCT is widely considered the reference standard for studies investigating the effect of one or more innovative or experimental treatments compared to the standard of care. An RCT can only be conducted, if there is therapeutic uncertainty (or equipoise) with regard to the variety of treatments available. The one and only key issue to the RCT is that it distributes both known and unknown confounders symmetrically to treatment arms, making the groups qualitatively similar. It thus allows for causal inferences on the effects of a certain treatment compared to controls. Whenever you have apparently comparable treatment alternatives available—aim for an RCT. It is the most simple and ethically justified study design you can imagine (see pages 21, 36, 38).

regression   Regression is a tool to explain how much of the variance of one variable is explained by another. There is a vast number of regression models for binary (eg, logistic), categorical (eg, ordinal logistic), and continuous data (eg, linear) available, and implemented in common statistical software packages like SPSS, SAS, and STATA. Some advice: it takes time and skills to do both meaningful unvariable and multivariable regression analyses. Leave this to your methodological consultant rather than doing them by your own—they are tricky and time consuming (see pages 108, 126, 127, 133).

relative risk (or risk ratio)   The risk of developing an event under a certain exposure or treatment divided by the risk of developing an event under another exposure or treatment (see pages 18, 23, 25, 28, 99).

risk difference   The risk of developing an event under a certain exposure or treatment minus the risk of developing an event under another exposure or treatment (see pages 26–28).

sample   A sample is a collection of units from a population willing to participate in your study. It is the best approximation to the population, since you cannot include all subjects hypothetically eligible for your study (see pages 8, 9, 12–15, 19, 27, 32, 40, 44, 45, 50, 51, 55, 72, 73, 78, 100, 105, 118, 126, 133).

significance   The significance level of a hypothesis test is the chance that the test erroneously rejects the null hypothesis when the null hypothesis is true. The widely accepted level of statistical significance is 5% (see *P* value), but this is a pragmatic convention rather than a biological constant. It also does not indicate whether observed differences are clinically meaningful (see pages 97, 99, 103, 104, 107, 118, 120, 134).

statistic   A number that is computed from data to compute *P* values. There is, of course, much more to learn about this process if you really want to. If not, be comfortable with the definition of a value derived from data that are used to investigate whether there is some chance that results have occurred by chance.

statistician   A statistician is a machine that transforms coffee into theorems (and, of course, your best and reliable friend when planning, conducting, and analyzing a clinical trial).

t-test   A classic hypothesis test for evaluating differences in mean values, when the distribution of values is known to be nearly normal (see pages 96–98, 104–107).

type I and type II errors   These refer to hypothesis testing. A type I error (or alpha error) occurs when the null hypothesis is rejected erroneously when it is in fact true. This means that, although there is no advantage of a treatment under investigation, the study suggests there is an advantage. To minimize the risk of applying treatments to patients that have falsely been tested positive in clinical studies, alpha is usually set at low levels like 5%. A type II error (or beta error) occurs if the null hypothesis is not rejected although there is an effect of the treatment under investigation. Typically, this happens if the study was not adequately powered, meaning that too small a number of patients had been recruited onto the trial (see pages 39–41).

variance   The variance of a list of numbers is the square of the standard deviation, that is the average of the squares of the deviations of the numbers in the list from their mean (see pages 96, 101, 106).

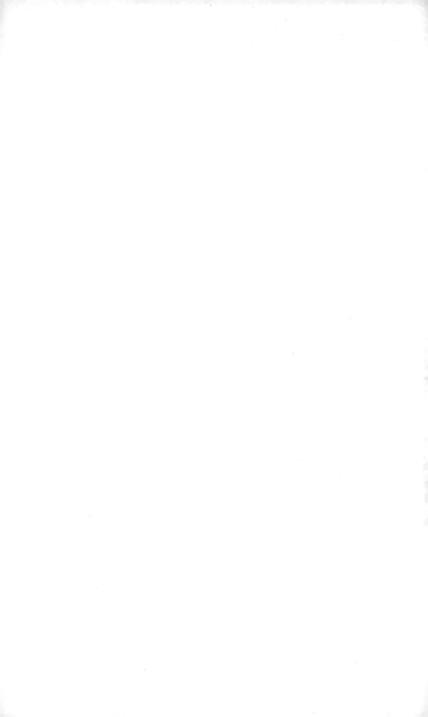